IN CHARGE OF THE WARD

In Charge of the Ward

Third Edition

ARLINE MATTHEWS

RGN DN (Univ. of London)
Clinical Nurse Specialist, Haematology,
Royal Hallamshire Hospital, Sheffield;
formerly Ward Sister, Royal Hallamshire Hospital, Sheffield

and

JANET WHELAN

BSc, RGN, MSc
formerly Macmillan Lecturer in Cancer Nursing,
The Royal Marsden Hospital, London

Blackwell Science

© 1982, 1987, 1993 by
Blackwell Science Ltd
Editorial Offices:
Osney Mead, Oxford OX2 0EL
25 John Street, London WC1N 2BL
23 Ainslie Place, Edinburgh EH3 6AJ
238 Main Street, Cambridge,
   Massachusetts 02142, USA
54 University Street, Carlton
   Victoria 3053, Australia

Other Editorial Offices:
Arnette Blackwell SA
1, rue de Lille
75007 Paris
France

Blackwell Wissenschafts-Verlag GmbH
Kurfürstendamm 57
10707 Berlin
Germany

Blackwell MZV
Feldgasse 13
A-1238 Wien
Austria

DISTRIBUTORS
Marston Book Services Ltd
PO Box 87
Oxford OX2 0DT
(*Orders:* Tel: 01865 791155
      Fax: 01865 791927
      Telex: 837515)

North America
Blackwell Science, Inc.
238 Main Street
Cambridge, MA 02142
(*Orders:* Tel: 800 215-1000
      617 876-7000
      Fax: 617 492-5263)

Australia
Blackwell Science Pty Ltd
54 University Street
Carlton, Victoria 3053
(*Orders:* Tel: 03 347-5552)

A catalogue record for this book is
available from the British Library

ISBN 0–632–03448–3

Library of Congress
Cataloging in Publication Data
is available

First published 1982
Reprinted 1984, 1985, 1986
Second edition 1987
Reprinted 1989, 1991
Third edition 1993
Reprinted 1995

Set by DP Photosetting Ltd, Aylesbury, Bucks
Printed and bound in Great Britain by
Biddles Ltd, Guildford and King's Lynn

Contents

Foreword by Dr Susan Pembrey   vii

Preface   ix

1   The role and functions of the ward sister or charge nurse   1

2   Communication   25

3   Taking on a new ward   41

4   Nursing research, computers in nursing, ward budgeting,   56
    presentation and analysis of data

5   Quality in nursing   78

6   Day-to-day organization in the ward   96

7   Preparation for inpatient care   137

8   The multidisciplinary team approach   159

9   Continuing care   178

10 Creating a high morale within the team   204

11 Teaching in the ward   215

12 The changing role of the nurse and the legal implications in   241
    patient care

    Appendix I   260

    Appendix II   263

    Appendix III   265

    Index   267

Foreword

If I was a newly-appointed ward sister I would regard this book as a true friend and one of my most useful possessions. It is written by one of the most experienced, able and caring sisters that I know and is a practical source of help for new ward sisters, who are usually expected to be founts of immediate knowledge and expertise. This book is a source of real wisdom born of many years of experience, clearly conveyed in these pages. It is this wisdom and true care for patients and staff that makes Arline Matthews special.

It is acknowledged in the preface that the once well-established role of the ward sister or charge nurse is now being challenged, and numerous changes are affecting it. Many of these changes are reflected in this expanded third edition, where Arline is joined by her collaborator Janet Whelan to give essential and helpful information on computers, ward budgeting, research, presentation of data and the rapidly developing field of quality assurance.

Behind these changes lies the core of the ward sister's work, the onerous professional responsibility for a human service of great creativity, subtlety and complexity: a service that could be undermined by some of the current changes if they go too far. Arline sets the right note by commenting 'I have continued to refer to the ward sister or charge nurse rather than the ward manager. After all, the patient knows who sister is; the ward manager could be anyone'.

Turn to the chapters on taking on a new ward, day-to-day organisation, continuing care, creating a high morale within the team, teaching in the ward; here you will find the unchanging heart of the ward sister's work and the particular contribution it makes. I recommend this wise and practical book.

Dr Susan Pembrey, OBE, FRCN, PhD
Senior Fellow, National Institute for Nursing
Radcliffe Infirmary, Oxford

Preface

The aim of this book when first written, was to help the newly appointed and less experienced ward sisters and charge nurses to prepare for their new role. The object was to help them by:

(1) Defining the role and giving guidance on the functions of the nurse in charge of the ward;
(2) Emphasizing the management aspects of the role in relation to the clinical aspects;
(3) Demonstrating the leadership aspects of the role;
(4) Building on the concepts of ward management learnt as part of the nurse education curriculum.

The book aims to provide a practical guide to the nurse taking charge of a ward. It should be possible to read it from cover to cover, to use it as a source of reference or to dip into it for specific information.

Ideally, all staff nurses should undertake a management course to prepare them for their new role. Unfortunately this is not always possible. The principles covered in this book may be applied to any ward or department whatever the specialty.

Preparing this third edition has been very difficult as the once-well-established role of the ward sister or charge nurse is being challenged. The role is being affected by the numerous changes taking place both structurally and functionally within the National Health Service – changes which are likely to continue for some time to come. Until now there has always been an acceptable balance between the clinical and managerial responsibilities within the role, but this balance is changing in favour of the managerial functions. The expectations are unrealistic, however, as all too often the sister or charge nurse is expected to carry out these extra functions within the current constraints, and still remain part of the rostered service.

It is apparent that the role of the ward sister or charge nurse will vary greatly from one hospital to another as the developments within the health service are interpreted differently. It must be remembered, however, that the making of a good ward sister or charge nurse depends to a large extent on the sound knowledge, skill and experience acquired following registration and before taking up the post. In order to demonstrate competence in the job, an understanding of the behaviour of individuals in stressful as well as normal circumstances must be shown.

This third edition includes two additional chapters which provide an introduction to some of the new activities which may take place within wards and departments. These reflect the changing role of the sister or charge nurse with a move towards greater managerial and teaching responsibilities.

Some critics will comment that I have not developed certain aspects of the role sufficiently, having retained some traditional views. I have attempted to take the middle line, always keeping in mind that in some wards the role will be far more developed than in others, but I do acknowledge that with on-going changes within the National Health Service the role will alter.

I would ask readers to look on *In Charge of the Ward* as a first book – an introduction to the role of the nurse in charge of the ward – which can be used as a stepping stone to more in-depth reading.

Although intended primarily for ward sisters and charge nurses I hope that this book will be of help to staff nurses, enrolled nurses – especially those undertaking a conversion course – and final-year student nurses.

In this edition the new health care worker is referred to as support worker and the reference to nursing officer has been changed to clinical nurse manager. I have continued to refer to the ward sister or charge nurse rather than the ward manager. After all, the patient knows who sister is; the ward manager could be anyone.

Arline Matthews
March 1993

Chapter 1
The role and functions of the ward sister or charge nurse

The role of the ward sister or charge nurse is unique. She or he is nearly always in charge of the ward when on duty, and holds responsibility for some aspects of the nursing actions that take place even when he or she is not there. He or she is usually the figurehead to whom everyone tends to turn. Those within the ward (the patients, nurses, doctors), those who visit (the relatives, visiting doctors), and many others, all look for the sister or charge nurse, expecting answers to their many queries. Even following days-off and annual leave, she or he is still expected to come up with all the answers! Research has shown that the sister or charge nurse can expect to be interrupted, on average, every six minutes! (Pembrey, 1980)

Sisters and charge nurses are expected to know how to cope with all situations and to know where to turn for advice, guidance or information if they don't have it themselves.

The Briggs Report (1972) stated:

> The ward or departmental sister is the key person there: her powers vary according to the administrative policy of the hospital... Her own personality is important in creating the atmosphere most conducive to happier nurses and patients...
>
> Most important of all, she has the power to affect the morale of the whole ward, more even than it is affected by the nature of the disease cared for in that ward... (p. 36)

Despite the changes in nursing and in the health service generally, this statement seems just as valid now as it did 20 years ago!

Since the time of the Briggs report, there has been much research into the work of the ward sister or charge nurse and the effect that this individual can have on the learner nurses, the staff's attitude to the work, their patients and their colleagues, and on the ward atmosphere generally (Perry, 1978; Orton, 1981; Fretwell, 1982; Ogier, 1982). Some of their findings – together with literature from other, related, areas such as sociology and management, and personal experience – are used to describe the role and functions of the ward sister in the rest of this chapter.

The demands made of the person in charge of the ward are daunting and seem to be never-ending – matched only by the extent of the influence that the ward sister or charge nurse has on all those he or she has contact with. It can be frightening to think that the leadership ability, attitudes, behaviour and moods of this key person can be so pervasive – but all the more important to look at the role in more detail, and to reflect on the many functions of the nurse in charge of the ward.

Webster's dictionary (1981) defines 'role' as 'a socially prescribed pattern of behaviour corresponding to an individual's status in a particular society'. Thus a ward sister or charge nurse's role can be seen as the behaviour that goes with that position – prescribed partly by the hospital, partly by the profession and partly by his or her colleagues, as well as by his or her own personal expectations and standards. It may take a newly appointed sister or charge nurse some time to develop the role to his or her satisfaction. Indeed, the role may change in time, as a result of influences outside as well as from personal and professional development of the individual. For example, a newly appointed sister or charge nurse may find difficulty in relating to staff nurses, enrolled nurses or support workers who are older; whereas, some patients and their relatives may have the same difficulty in reverse. If the appropriate behaviour that is expected of the position is adopted, respect and confidence from others will be won. Those appointed to the post in the same hospital where they were staff nurses, especially if on the same ward, may find it particularly difficult.

Behaviour pattern (Fig. 1.1)

The attitude adopted to patients, their relatives and staff is most important as first impressions have a far-reaching effect. The behaviour pattern will include:

(1) Setting a good example
(2) Knowing patients and staff
(3) Being available and approachable
(4) Being consistent
(5) Showing compassion and being perceptive of the needs of others
(6) Being receptive to the ideas of others
(7) Showing competence as a nurse

These will each be addressed in more detail.

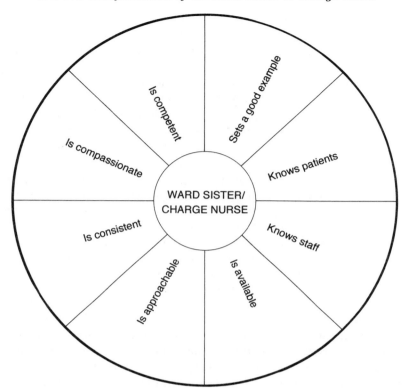

Fig. 1.1　The behaviour pattern of the ward sister/charge nurse.

Setting a good example

The sister or charge nurse is on show to patients, their relatives, and staff for the whole span of duty. The way people are spoken to and the way work is carried out will be observed by others and accepted as the correct way to act. Nurse learners and staff will learn from the sister or charge nurse's behaviour, and others will make judgements about the standards exhibited. So it is important that the correct messages are sent by behaving in an appropriate way. This means adhering to hospital policy and procedures at all times.

It is also important to consider the impact of the 'look' of the nurse in charge as many people will infer competence from this. The nurse must be aware of the image that she projects and feel happy that it conforms with her role. The debate about uniform for nurses continues, but whatever her opinion, the nurse must adhere to hospital policy and ensure that her make-up, hair style and jewellery are appropriate to the setting.

Knowing patients and staff

Getting to know patients' and colleagues' names will involve making an effort, especially on return from days-off or annual leave, but it is worth it as it makes each individual feel more at ease and cared about. If a name is difficult to pronounce it is important to make a special effort to use it correctly; ask the person concerned how to pronounce it if necessary. It is always a good idea to ask patients and colleagues by what name they like to be addressed – and then use it. Some older people do not like the common use of first names.

A nurse should never refer to the patient as 'the appendix in bed 4' or 'the patient with the cholecystectomy'. Thinking and speaking of patients as individual human beings will influence the attitude of other members of the ward team too.

Walking onto a ward for the first time, a nurse may feel very nervous and apprehensive. If addressed by name, the nurse will begin to feel a little more at ease, knowing that the arrival of a new nurse is thoughtfully anticipated. The same attitude applies to patients.

Being available and approachable

Always managing to smile, even when the going gets hard, helps most patients and makes the sister or charge nurse appear approachable and understanding. A smile indicates that a person is happy, and patients have said that it makes a difference to the way they feel in hospital if they know that the nurses caring for them are happy.

The ward sister or charge nurse should aim to appear available to patients, their relatives and the staff, and never be remote. Those who are approachable at all times, and willing to listen, gain the confidence and respect of both patients and staff. It is important to remember that everyone needs to talk in depth at times, and a willingness to listen will often encourage this.

To be available and approachable to patients' relatives it is necessary to go to meet them and not wait for them to come to you. Many relatives are afraid to go and seek information, especially if it means knocking on the office door.

Working with the nurses and actively showing an interest in what they are doing will ensure that the sister or charge nurse is available to them. The way in which a nurse receives an answer to questions will demonstrate whether the sister or charge nurse is approachable. Face-to-face contact is also a good indicator.

Spending time with every patient at the beginning of the span of duty is helpful if the sister or charge nurse is to ensure approachability. In addition it provides an opportunity to:

(1)   Assess each patient's needs
(2)   Assess the state of the ward
(3)   Assess the nursing workload
(4)   Enable the patients to ask questions
(5)   Give and receive information from patients and their relatives
(6)   Assess the need for nurse education and support, both for individual nurses and for the entire nursing team.

As long as the nurse in charge does not give the impression of being in a hurry or of being an inspector, a round of the patients gives them and their nurses an opportunity to voice anxieties and fears.

Being consistent

The nurse in charge should be consistent in mood and never up one day and down the next so that neither staff nor the patients know where they are. Consistency in decision-making, behaviour and attitude to patients and colleagues must be demonstrated, and maturity in all matters – never childishness – will instil confidence. The sister or charge nurse should not allow personal worries to affect work. If personal problems are 'brought to work' these will often reflect on the staff and also make the sister or charge nurse inconsistent in the performance of duty.

Consistency between what is taught by teachers of nurses and what is practised in the ward is essential. In other words, the ideas of those in the nursing service should match those of nurse educators.

This may be done by:

(1)   Ensuring all nurses know what is expected of them when they come to the ward
(2)   Carrying out procedures correctly, following accepted principles based on agreed standards of care
(3)   Being available to advise, support, supervise and guide nurses on the ward
(4)   Ensuring good two-way communication between the teachers and the ward
(5)   Ensuring that the philosophy of nursing used on the ward supports and supplements the philosophy of nurse education.

Showing compassion and being perceptive

A good ward sister or charge nurse must be perceptive of the needs of both patients and staff, and show compassion. A compassionate approach is one which shows an understanding of the position of others and a willingness to help them. The sister or charge nurse needs to show an understanding of the psychological and emotional needs of patients, their relatives, and staff, and must always be able to put herself or himself in the place of others to appreciate how they feel in a particular situation.

Being receptive to the ideas of others

Receptivity to suggestions made by the nurses, allowing all to participate and contribute their ideas, is another mark of a good sister or charge nurse. If a nurse questions what is being done, this is looked on as a positive and constructive approach and not as a matter of one being impertinent or insubordinate. Too frequently nurses in training have been classed as 'difficult' or 'troublemakers' if they questioned established practices, and this sort of labelling can only bring harm to the profession. A questioning attitude is a positive and healthy approach, and helps to keep the permanent members of the ward team on their toes and up-to-date.

The sister or charge nurse needs to be forward-thinking and willing to innovate with sufficient self-confidence to feel not threatened by but rather receptive to other people's ideas or suggestions. The ward philosophy, routine and methods of working must be continually reappraised and reassessed. This must be done with an open mind and constructive self-criticism in order not to become outdated and entrenched in one's own ways to the exclusion of all others. In brief, a sister or charge nurse cannot afford to slip into a 'rut'. Attitudes must be flexible – but not flaccid – and the methods and ideas employed must reflect this flexibility.

Showing competence as a nurse

The ward sister or charge nurse must be a competent nurse and personally able to give a high standard of care, demonstrating ability through in-depth knowledge of nursing and, in particular, the speciality, in discussions about patients' needs. This kind of competence should also be apparent when explaining to nurses the reasons for certain nursing and medical actions.

In day-to-day contact with patients and nurses there are many opportunities to show expertise, such as:

● Showing a nurse how to position a patient comfortably
● Teaching a nurse how to give an injection proficiently

- Demonstrating the technique for performing a difficult, painful dressing
- Demonstrating the correct administration of drugs
- Talking to distressed relatives.

The way in which the ward sister or charge nurse sees and interprets the role can be observed in all these aspects of his or her behaviour. But 'being in charge of the ward' is not just about adopting certain behaviour: the ward sister or charge nurse must function effectively as manager, leader, teacher, co-ordinator, worker, supervisor and friend, to mention but a few aspects.

One reason why so many things are asked of a ward sister or charge nurse is that many people are involved in the proper functioning of a ward. It is not just nursing tasks that are undertaken there; there is a continuing presence of medical staff, ward pharmacists, ancillary staff, and so on. They will all demand some acknowledgement from the ward sister or charge nurse and disrupt the flow of the nursing work. A happy ward depends on the relationships within the multidisciplinary team and with all the departments within the hospital, recognizing that all have a vital role to play, even when not directly involved in patient care.

The nursing team itself is, of course, also made up of individuals, each with unique needs for support, education and development. As the nursing team changes – often as frequently as weekly - the ward sister or charge nurse must continually assess the needs of the nurses and adapt his or her functioning accordingly.

The effectiveness with which all these functions are achieved will, to a certain extent, depend on an ability to develop managerial skills, the concepts of which will have been learnt as a staff nurse. Management is about working with people and getting things done well.

In general terms, the ward sister or charge nurse's main aim is to create a ward atmosphere and environment in which patients receive a high level of nursing care – every aspect of which is effectively and competently provided and co-ordinated with the care given by other professionals. The rest of this chapter looks at some aspects of the management and leadership skills required by the nurse in charge of a ward which enable him or her to attain this aim.

Figure 1.2 illustrates the ward sister or charge nurse's cycle of management and emphasizes the importance of communication and interaction for effective functioning. For this reason, the topic of communication is discussed in detail in the next chapter. Figure 1.2 provides the framework for addressing the functions of the ward sister or charge nurse in the rest of this chapter. These are:

(1) Leading
(2) Planning and organizing
(3) Prescribing
(4) Delegating
(5) Coordinating
(6) Supervising and directing
(7) Encouraging and supporting
(8) Caring and counselling
(9) Teaching and training
(10) Appraising and disciplining.

Leadership

Leadership is a vital part of the function of the ward sister or charge nurse. It establishes what kind of morale is created within the team.

Perry (1978) believes that:

A friendly happy atmosphere is particularly noticeable on a ward where the ward sister is a good leader. The atmosphere is noticed by the patients and contributes to their confidence in the staff, thus

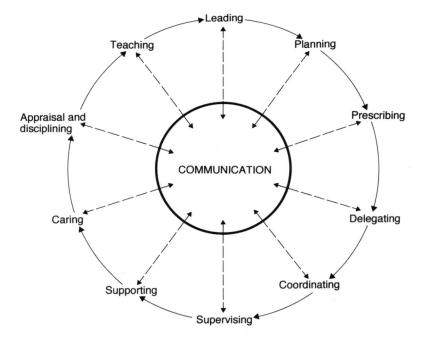

Fig. 1.2 The ward sister/charge nurse's cycle of management. All the functions are based on interaction

helping them to respond to treatment. In such a ward, the general standard of nursing care is good and is maintained in sister's absence.

There has been considerable research into leadership styles and skills in industry and organizations, as well as within health service settings. It is not possible to provide adequate cover of all the research findings here, but for those who are interested in pursuing the topic, there is a recommended reading list at the end of the chapter. It seems that the order prevailing on a ward is the outcome of complex relationships. The order is rooted in traditions, rules, and routines, but it is changed by an individual's negotiations within and outside the ward. The leadership style prevalent on the ward plays an important part in determining the relative importance of each of these factors. Lewin, Lipitt and White (1939) identified three styles of leadership, namely:

- Laissez-faire – leaders make minimal contact with and have minimal influence over subordinates
- Directive or autocratic – leaders in close contact with subordinates influence their actions, but are not, in turn, influenced by them
- Participative or democratic – leaders characterized as having frequent contact with subordinates and being strongly influenced by them.

These categories have been used extensively since 1939, and it has been found that the most effective managerial style is that exhibited by democratic leaders.

Other studies have used different classifications of management style and commonly it has been found that managers who are considerate of their subordinates and responsive to their needs produce good results. Equally, those who place high importance on getting the job done, and ensure that the environment and facilities are available to achieve that end, also make good leaders.

Although the style of leadership that gets the best from people is the democratic one – placing importance on the individual's needs as well as on getting the job done – leadership style must be flexible and will vary according to the situation. As the figure of authority with patients, visitors and staff, it is the sister or charge nurse who maintains discipline and order in the ward.

Planning and organizing

Planning involves giving forethought and consideration to any action and then making the necessary arrangements to carry out that action in the best possible way. Careful planning is essential so that time is not wasted, and also so that all staff are used to their full potential. Remember, the most precious resources which the sisters and charge nurses have at their disposal are people and time.

There are long-term plans that may take months or years to come to fruition, and immediate plans for the day-to-day running of the ward. Long-term plans might include such things as the development of a folder of literature, information and research articles which are relevant to the ward and to be used by students or new staff to increase their knowledge base in a speciality. More immediate plans might include the assignment of staff – taking into consideration the needs of the patients and the skills of the available staff. Immediate plans might also include ensuring that equipment and supplies are ready and available for use as they are needed. Intermediate plans include things like doing the duty rotas.

A positive way of ensuring that the plans are carried through and the organization of the ward is efficient, is to discuss the plans with the ward team so that everyone is able to pull in the same direction. Methods of ward organization and other aspects of planning are examined in Chapters 5 and 10.

Prescribing

Although the doctor prescribes the medical or surgical treatment for a patient, it is the registered general nurse who prescribes the nursing care. Problems are identified, and then a plan of care is developed based on the needs of each patient. Whenever possible, the patient or relatives should be consulted and involved. Although the registered general nurse is trained to prescribe and plan care, the sister's or charge nurse's knowledge and expertise should complement this, and she or he is available to guide and support. The sister or charge nurse must encourage the trained nurses to develop and perfect this approach to patient care. Remember, the nurse in charge is usually held accountable for the care prescribed and administered to each patient.

In some situations prescribing care requires discussion with the doctor: for example, the mobilization of a patient following certain surgical procedures; bowel care when a prescription for an aperient may be indicated; the giving of certain information to patients or their relatives which may overlap with medical information; or the arrangement of a suitable date for discharge. The need for team-work cannot be overemphasized.

Delegating

Delegation of responsibility is one of the most difficult aspects of a ward sister's or charge nurse's job. It is very tempting, on first being appointed, to assume total responsibility for the running of the ward and care of the patients. This is possibly because of a lack of self-confidence (or of confidence in others) and a desire to show an ability to cope with the job.

Delegation means entrusting authority, and with it responsibility for decision-making, to another, but the person who delegates always remains accountable. Before delegating, the sister or charge nurse must be fully conversant with the role and abilities of each nursing member of the ward team. (See Chapters 3 and 11). If the sister or charge nurse or any trained nurse knowingly delegates care to another nurse who has not the knowledge, skill or necessary training, she or he stands accountable for any errors or problems which occur. The outcome could be tragic.

Delegation is not a means of passing on jobs that are disliked, although it does spread the workload whilst ensuring coordination of effort.

If care is delegated, and with it the responsibility of ensuring that the patient receives a high standard of care, it is a way of ensuring that others:

- Are aware of what is expected of them
- Develop their ability, use their judgement and make decisions
- Have an opportunity to use their ideas
- Gain a sense of responsibility
- Gain job satisfaction
- Feel secure in the ward team.

It is important to delegate appropriately, and having done so, to allow team members to carry out their tasks, giving support or education if necessary.

If time is spent performing jobs that can or should be done by others, such as completing bed statements, filling in laboratory request forms, obtaining laboratory or X-ray results, ordering ambulances, booking appointments, preparing equipment for procedures or making coffee for doctors, valuable time is wasted. Little time will be left for the important aspects of the job.

Harmony and a good working relationship within the ward are maintained when the nursing team know that the sister or charge nurse trusts them and is loyal to them; this is best shown in the way that care and responsibility are delegated to the team members and they are allowed to proceed without interruptions. By delegating to the team members, the nurse in charge will be more available to guide, supervise, support and teach within the ward.

How do you delegate?

(1)　Ensure that the nurse has the ability to deliver the necessary care at the required standard.

(2)　Ensure that the nurse knows what she or he is to do.

(3)　Make each nurse answerable for the care she or he has given and allow time to report back, to evaluate the care, and to alter any care plans (doing so eliminates the need to check up on the nurse). This can be termed allowing time for *feedback*.

Although the term *feedback* is basically computer jargon it is being used more frequently in nursing to demonstrate that information is fed back to the ward sister or charge nurse by the nurses delivering patient care. It is one of the ways in which information is obtained about the patients – their progress, their reaction to hospitalization, their concern about their family, their worries about impending treatment, and so forth. By showing a receptiveness to this detailed information and taking appropriate action as indicated, the sister or charge nurse demonstrates that the contribution of each team member is valued regardless of their seniority.

If an official time is set aside each day for the passing on of information, the sister or charge nurse ensures that the nurses remain answerable for the care given by them. It also gives an opportunity to share information gained with other health care workers.

The nurses also need to receive feedback. This includes information about their patients and also how they themselves are getting on in their work.

(4)　When something or someone needs urgent attention approach the nurse caring for the patient and not the first nurse at hand, even if this is quicker and easier, unless it is an emergency situation.

(5)　Do not do the job yourself, even if it is quicker than teaching the nurse, and do not delegate an activity and then carry out the job. This will undermine the nurse's confidence.

(6)　Allow the nurses to get on with planning and giving care, and do not continually check up. This also means allowing them to assess their priorities for care.

(7)　When care has been delegated:

- give guidance
- give support
- be available to the nurse

(8) Remain accountable if the new nurse is unqualified.
(9) Give final approval. If nursing care or any task is delegated, the person who delegates must always follow-up and ensure that the care has been given to the required standard. In the case of a task such as completion of the duty rota, final approval must be given. Delegation must never be followed by abdication of responsibility.

What can be delegated?

When delegating total care, it should be stressed that everything required by that patient is given by the nurse responsible for the patient's care. This will include general hygiene and comfort, care of the wound, administration of routine and 'as required' drugs. It should also include writing the progress report, giving the patient explanations about tests, and discussing discharge arrangements. However, when care is delegated to learner nurses they will need a certain amount of supervision, depending on their stage of training, previous experience and level of knowledge.

Specific responsibilities can be given to permanent team members. This is referred to as functional delegation. The sister or charge nurse is responsible for ensuring that these activities are carried out, but she or he must allow the nurses to get on with their work and not continually check up on them.

Accountability

The ward sister or charge nurse is accountable for her or his actions, and responsible for the practice delegated to the unqualified members of the team, i.e. student/learner nurses, support workers or nursing auxiliaries being responsible for whatever they do. The trained nurses in the team, however, are responsible for their own actions and are held accountable for the standard of care and everything they provide, or omit to give or do. The trained nurse must work within the limits of her or his professional competence, and is responsible for what she or he has been directed to do, e.g. planning care for a group of patients, but she or he is held accountable for the care assessed, planned and given, by explaining the rationale for all decisions made by her or him.

The trained nurse has a duty of care and is accountable to the patient, his or her relatives, society, the profession and the health service, and she or he may be called to explain and defend her or his actions and decisions, basing argument on sound professional knowledge and judgement. The UKCC Code of Professional Conduct (see Chapter 12 and Appendix 1) instructs nurses to exercise responsibility and judgement and to always act in the best interests of the patient, and be accountable for decisions they make about patient care.

Coordinating

Coordination is bringing everything together so that every element is in proper relationship with each other, and as the ward sister or charge nurse is seen as the key figure, she or he is the obvious person to coordinate all the activities within the ward.

These include:

- Delivery of patient care
- Activities of the nursing team
- Activities of the multidisciplinary health care team
- Information coming into the ward
- Ward services.

The sister or charge nurse must coordinate the delivery of care to the patients throughout the day, ensuring that all the nursing staff work together as a team and pull in the same direction to ensure that the provision of patient care runs smoothly. If each nurse, or team of nurses went their own way without any thought for the rest of the ward and no-one coordinated the whole, chaos would occur, especially in an emergency.

There must be close liaison between the sister or charge nurse and the nurses. Proper coordination is based on sound planning and the cooperation of others. The coordinator must be available, continually circulating amongst patients and staff, encouraging them and keeping them informed of changes and new developments. As the coordinator of activities within the ward, the sister or charge nurse must be kept informed by the nurses when doctors or other health workers are contacted, so that they are not disturbed unnecessarily. If the doctor, for example, has already been asked to come to the ward to see a patient, it is pointless to contact him or her again to come to see another patient, unless it is urgent. Close liaison with the doctors is very important. Coordination between the doctors and the nurses responsible for the care of the patients is essential so that the doctors are aware of changes in a patient's condition.

Many health care workers, such as social workers, community nurses, or physiotherapists, can be involved in the patients' care and it will often fall to the ward sister or charge nurse to coordinate these services, ensuring they are informed of changes, exchanging relevant information, and linking them with the nurses giving the care.

To coordinate successfully, she or he needs to understand and respect the role of other health workers, and ensure that the ward nurses are also aware of the role of others.

In order that the ward runs smoothly, there has to be close liaison between the sister or charge nurse and the ward clerk or secretary who receives much of the information coming into the ward, especially telephoned information. The sister or charge nurse has to decide whether to act on the information herself, allow the ward clerk to take action, or direct the ward clerk to pass it onto a third person who may be the doctor, nurse or one of the other health care workers.

Another area requiring coordination, is that of various services such as supplies of drugs, equipment, linen, dressings, etc., in order that these are available at the right time and at the correct levels so that activities in the ward can run smoothly. This will mean liaising and cooperating with members of other departments, planning ahead with them, and making sure that orders are put in at the right time. This may be daily or weekly, depending on the department concerned and the particular hospital.

Today there is a tendency towards 'topping-up' systems, especially with drug supplies and central sterile supplies. This means that a member of staff from the department concerned brings the ward stock of items issued by that department up to a predetermined level. This level is discussed and agreed beforehand by a member of the department and the ward sister or charge nurse.

There must still be some nursing input and control, especially before week-ends and bank holidays, when a check of stock levels will need to be made to make sure that stocks of essential items will not run out. From time to time, the sister or charge nurse will need to review the stock levels, and if they are inappropriate, arrangements should be made with the department concerned for the levels to be increased or decreased.

Supervising and directing

Supervision is, or should be, a democratic process during which the nurses are given every help and encouragement by the ward sister or charge nurse. It is a method by which the nurses are helped to perform their work and give patient care safely and competently because their performance is being measured or monitored continually by the sister or charge nurse, who must ensure that the job is being done correctly, to the highest possible standard and within the agreed ward philosophy of care. It is not a means of checking up on each nurse and finding fault, but is a constructive exercise in which each nurse is enabled to develop his or her caring role and expertise. The supervisor must recognize the value of each member of the team and that each one has a vital part to play in achieving a high level of patient care and an atmosphere of high morale. A supervisor is not a person who always gives orders and directions but does not work.

Kron (1987) summarizes supervision in a most meaningful way, bringing in all the facets of a democratic supervisor as shown in Fig. 1.3.

In order to supervise effectively, the ward sister or charge nurse should be readily available. If heavily involved in nursing activities, such as bathing patients, dressing wounds or assisting with procedures, it is not possible to be readily available to supervise and teach the nursing team. This is why it is essential for the nurse in charge of the ward to delegate.

The sister or charge nurse supervises the nursing personnel, nursing care and other activities in the ward. Some of these activities have been taken over by ancillary staff or contract workers in some hospitals, but nursing input is still required. An obvious example is the serving of patients' meals. Ensuring that patients receive the diets that they require, presented in an appealing way is a nurse's responsibility and monitoring a patient's intake of food may be a part of the prescribed nursing care.

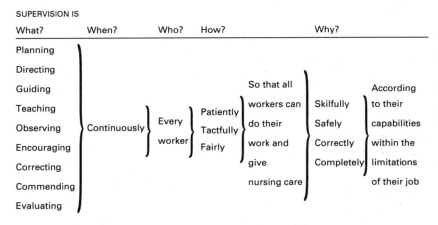

Fig. 1.3 Kron's summary of supervision.

Meals are very important to most patients and should be recognized as such by the nurses and not just seen as another chore to be got through as quickly as possible.

The sister or charge nurse directs nursing care. This forms part of the supervisory role. It involves guiding each nurse and ensuring that each one knows what to do and how to do it. Once care is delegated to each nurse, supervision and guidance is given by the sister or charge nurse when indicated. Directions are both written and verbal, involving detailed communication, and it is essential that the directions are understood by the nurses.

Encouraging and supporting

All nurses need encouragement so that they may fulfil their role and give nursing care – physical, psychological and spiritual care. Encouragement can be given in several ways:

- Giving thanks
- Giving praise
- Delegating effectively
- Allowing others to put forward their ideas.

Thanks and praise for work done are forms of encouragement. A nurse who has coped well with a difficult problem, working hard and competently, or comforting distressed relatives of a patient and giving them support during the terminal stages of a patient's illness, needs to know that this contribution has been appreciated. A nurse whose attitude to work has been a problem and, following discussion with the sister or charge nurse shows an improvement, should know that this has been noticed. Telling the nurse is an encouragement.

By delegating the care of patients to the nurses, the sister or charge nurse encourages them because they are given an opportunity to gain personal satisfaction in their work. When nurses are encouraged by the sister or charge nurse to contribute their ideas and suggestions, and they sense a receptiveness to their ideas, they will feel that they are valuable members of the ward team. By inviting their suggestions and allowing the nurses to put them into practice, the sister or charge nurse will be giving encouragement as well as support. To give their best, people need to feel the support of those around them and, in particular, of their superiors.

The ward sister or charge nurse gives support to the ward team by:

- Making them aware of her or his expectations
- Ensuring team members are kept well informed
- Assisting others to make decisions
- Giving advice
- Giving guidance
- Listening and giving explanations.

By advising and guiding the team, the ward sister or charge nurse gives support. By allowing the nurses to draw on her or his valuable experience when they are caring for their patients, the sister or charge nurse will be giving them solid support in their day-to-day responsibilities.

The ward sister or charge nurse provides emotional support for patients, their relatives and the nurses by listening and talking with them, giving explanations, answering their questions and sharing their problems and worries. Patients need explanations in order to prepare for what is to happen to them. These explanations include information about special investigations, drugs, all that is involved in having an operation and what to expect postoperatively. The patients need reassurance that if there is likely to be pain and discomfort it will be relieved, in order to minimize fear of the unknown. The nurse caring for the patient may prefer that these explanations are given by the more knowledgeable and experienced nurse in charge.

Relatives of a patient frequently need an interpretation into layman's terms of what the doctor has told them, and they will also want to discuss the patient's progress and plans for discharge. If this is readily available to them they will feel supported. Other health care professionals, such as the social worker or district nurse, may need to be included in these plans. The patient will almost certainly be included. Showing that one cares, by sharing joy or grief and sorrow, helps to give strength and is supportive.

Discussion with a nurse, following a difficult situation in the ward, will help the nurse to understand and prepare for similar situations in the future and, whilst in the ward, to feel a gaining of support from the sister or charge nurse. Encouraging the nurses to open up and discuss together how they feel about a particularly difficult problem, so that they become aware that others feel the same, is seen as being supportive.

Jennifer is 35 years old and aware that she is dying of lymphoma. She was extremely angry but is now coping with the support of husband, family, friends, doctors and nurses. A student nurse is finding it very difficult to relate to Jennifer because she identifies with her, but after talking about her feelings of anger and distress with the other ward nurses she finds that she can cope better herself and builds up a strong, helping relationship with Jennifer.

An additional sense of support is achieved if the sister or charge nurse explains why medical treatment is changed or stopped and the reasoning behind any nursing decisions made.

Caring and counselling

By showing empathy, love and compassion to patients, their relatives and staff, caring becomes apparent. Empathy is the capacity to put oneself in the position of others, demonstrating a real insight into what they are experiencing and seeing things as they do.

Counselling is helping a person to explore all aspects of a problem as a basis for deciding how to solve or cope with it. Members of the nursing team will look to the sister or charge nurse for assistance with a variety of issues and they will often need to talk through seemingly 'unfair' situations.

In stressful situations, what is usually required is a sister or charge nurse who will sit and listen while the nurse talks things through and reasons them out. Often the nurse will come to terms with the problem after thinking it through and may then be able to relate better to similar situations in the future.

The sister or charge nurse will also need to spend time listening to the patients and their relatives discussing their problems and worries. They need to be allowed to talk about how they will manage at home with what may be a completely new aspect of life such as coping with the loss of a spouse or loved one, altered life expectancy, alteration in body image such as learning to live with a colostomy or a breast prosthesis. Obviously, this counselling will be in addition to the practical support which must be provided and will also be given by the patient's own nurse and often other health care workers.

Caring means showing concern for and taking an interest in a person. Care extends to patients, their relatives, and staff. When there is no interest and concern shown for the nursing team, the sister or charge nurse cannot expect them to care for their patients or show any interest in the set aims and objectives of the ward.

When caring for patients, one must consider total needs and not just those associated with the reason for their admission to hospital. One of the most important responsibilities is emphasizing to the nurses that to give a high level of care to their patients they must firstly recognize each patient as an individual and, secondly, that each individual has unique physical, psychological and spiritual needs.

Despite the effectiveness of example and skill, because of the managerial and supportive role, the sister or charge nurse may not be able to give much direct physical care to the patients. Nursing care is usually delegated, the sister or charge nurse providing supervision and support to the nursing team. Care and concern for patients and relatives can be demonstrated if the sister or charge nurse shows an understanding of the effect of illness and hospitalization on them and the different ways in which both patients and their relatives react to these circumstances.

The nursing team will be aware that the sister or charge nurse cares for them if she or he shows an awareness of their needs – their need for support, encouragement, advice, job satisfaction, education and training, a varied experience and a sense of responsibility.

Teaching and training

As teaching is a vital aspect of the function of the ward sister or charge nurse it will be covered fully in Chapter 11. This aspect of the work involves teaching and training all staff involved with the ward – nurses, support workers, ancillary staff – and patients and their relatives.

All nurses have a right to know what is expected of them – what they are to do and how they must perform. In a ward where emphasis is placed on teaching and training, a good name is gained by that ward and good morale tends to be maintained. It is usually a ward where nurses are attracted back once they have qualified.

If time is taken and effort made to fully orientate a new trained nurse to the ward, explaining the philosophy and how the ward is organized, the new member should smoothly join the team. If trained staff are orientated well the ward should run efficiently at all times. The effective training of the already trained nurses will also involve delegating to them some responsibility for running the ward when the sister or charge nurse is on duty, so that they gain confidence and experience. This could include doctors' ward rounds, liaising with other departments and personnel, ordering of supplies, nurses' reports and contacting patients' relatives. The sister or charge nurse can act as adviser and guide to the nurse concerned.

While the teaching and training of ancillary staff is not the direct responsibility of the nurse in charge of the ward, he or she must recognize when a need for teaching or training exists, and, on occasion, provide special information relating to the ward or to a particular patient. Teaching does not always mean a formal teaching situation. The sister or charge nurse is always teaching by example. Many things cannot be taught in the classroom, only in the ward. A nurse can only learn how to answer the telephone efficiently or talk to the distressed relatives of patients by observing someone who is very experienced in this, and then putting these observations into practice.

Appraising and discipline

Nurses have a right to know what is expected of them and how well they are meeting these expectations. Most health authorities now have a policy or system for staff appraisal, the purpose of which is to:

(1) Increase the contribution of individual nurses in their current job
(2) Develop their potential abilities to meet the needs of the service of the future. (National Staff Committee (Nurses and Midwives) (1977).

It does not have as one of its objectives the notion of staff reward, nor is it to be seen as an opportunity for reprimand. The value of appraisal is the opportunity it provides for an open, purposeful and confidential discussion about the staff member's performance over an agreed period of time. Attention must be given to the whole range of activities for which the nurse has some responsibility, and the outcome of the interview should be the joint development of planned targets for the next review period.

In addition, the appraisal provides a formal opportunity for the ward sister or charge nurse to ask for feedback about how he or she has helped or hindered the staff. In receiving this feedback, it must be remembered that the person providing it may feel very uneasy about doing so, and may have limited experience in dealing with such situations, so it may not 'come out' in the way intended. It is important to receive feedback in a constructive and not a hostile way.

All nurses in training on the wards have their nursing abilities assessed on an ongoing basis. Ward sisters and charge nurses should take the opportunity to develop their skills as trainers and assessors in a more formal way (for example, ENB course 998 'Teaching and Assessing in Clinical Practice') if it is available, as they are going to be asked to do more and more assessment in clinical settings as the development of courses for care assistants progresses.

Appraisal and assessment are not the same thing, but the opportunity offered by continuous assessment during a nurse's allocation to the ward can be viewed as similar to an appraisal interview (see Chapter 11).

It is also the ward sister or charge nurse's responsibility to deal with disciplinary matters, in the first instance. The local disciplinary and grievance procedure should be laid down in full, and the ward sister or charge nurse must be familiar with it before taking any disciplinary action. Any nurse involved in a disciplinary procedure should be advised to consult her trade union or professional representative straight away. Whether the situation merits the full disciplinary procedure or merely some timely guidance, it should be done privately and as soon as possible after the incident has occurred. The interview must be conducted in a friendly, constructive manner and two-way communication is imperative so that the nurse involved feels that he or she has had a fair hearing.

Joint Appointments

An increasing number of sister or charge nurse posts are joint education/ service appointments, giving dual responsibility to the person in post. These posts may be ward sister/nurse tutor, ward sister/university lecturer, clinical nurse manager/nurse tutor. Some posts include a commitment to research.

The joint appointee is based in a clinical setting, but she or he has a definite teaching commitment within the nurse education centre, polytechnic or university. When away from the ward or department, she or he still remains responsible clinically and professionally, but this responsibility is usually shared with a second sister or charge nurse, or a senior staff nurse.

It has been found that joint appointment posts give more credibility to the appointees as nurse educators, as they have daily contact with patients and remain practitioners, thus helping to integrate education and service. They have a direct influence on what is taught in the nurse education centre or nursing department as they are able to keep up-to-date in both education and nursing practice.

Where there are two ward sisters or charge nurses on a ward, it is important for them to communicate well together to ensure that they provide complementary leadership styles. If conflicts between them arise, it can be detrimental to the entire ward team. Dividing the responsibilities so that each has a defined role can be a solution to the problem of conflict (Whelan, 1988).

The many functions of the ward sister or charge nurse are interrelated, making the job a very complex one. It is not an easy position to take on and much thought and effort must go into making the position effective and successful.

Topics for discussion

1. The effect of inconsistency in style and mood:

> When the ward was busy, an inexperienced sister kept making decisions about the management of the ward and within minutes would change her mind. She

would delegate care to the nurses one day and allow them to proceed freely with their plans. Another day, she would again delegate, but then interfere in the care. Sometimes she would be very friendly with all the nurses, while at others she would shout at them because their method of working did not coincide with hers.

Consider what effects this inexperienced sister would have on her team of nurses and suggest reasons why she might be exhibiting such inconsistent behaviour.

2. How to delegate:
Consider the following sequence of events:

An inexperienced sister, having asked a staff nurse to refer two of the patients allocated to her to the district nurse and write the appropriate letters, did so herself whilst the staff nurse was at lunch. She said she did so because she felt that the staff nurse would never do it.

How would this type of behaviour affect the staff nurse in the future? What effect could it have on the nursing team? What repercussions could it have for the ward sister?

3. Ward learning climate:

A nurse working on her first ward was made to feel that her observations of her patients and the reporting to the sister of information relating to them, gained whilst she was giving care, was regarded as of significance. However, on her next ward when she told sister that Mrs Fern, an elderly lady with a newly formed colostomy, would prefer to go to her own home instead of to the convalescent home as arranged, the sister gave her the impression that it was no concern of hers (the nurse) and virtually ignored the request.

Contrast the feedback and self-esteem gained by this nurse on each of these two wards and the effects it would have on the care given by her.

4. Discuss the issues that might be raised and identify the potential counselling needs for ward staff when the following things happen to patients on the ward:

(a) A patient has a medical abortion in a ward where there are also patients who are being investigated for infertility.
(b) The mother of three young children who is terminally ill is talking about the fact that she realizes that she will not see her children grow up.
(c) The only child of a widow dies of leukaemia.

References

Department of Health and Social Security, Scottish Home and Health Department, and Welsh Office (1972) *Report of the Committee on Nursing* (chairman A. Briggs), HMSO, London.

Fretwell, J.E. (1982) *Ward Teaching and Learning*, Royal College of Nursing, London.

Kron, T. (1987) *The Management of Nursing Care – putting leadership skills to work* (6th ed), Saunders Co., Philadelphia.

Lewin, K, Lipitt, R. and White, R.K. (1939) Patterns of aggressive behaviour in experimentally created social climates. *Journal of Social Psychology*, **10**, 271–99.

National Staff Committee (Nurses and Midwives) (1977) NHS Staff Development and Performance Review – Nurses, Midwives, Health Visitors and Tutorial Staff, DHSS.

Ogier, M.E. (1982) *An Ideal Sister?*, Royal College of Nursing, London.

Orton, H.D. (1981) *Ward Learning Climate*, Royal College of Nursing, London.

Pembrey, S. (1980) *The Ward Sister – Key to Nursing*, Royal College of Nursing, London.

Perry, E.L. (1978) *Ward Management and Teaching*, Ballière-Tindall, London.

Webster's Third New International Dictionary (1981), Encyclopaedia Britannica Inc., Chicago, USA.

Whelan, J. (1988) Ward Sisters' management styles and their effects on nurses' perceptions of quality of care. *Journal of Advanced Nursing*, **13**, 125–38.

Recommended Reading

Joint Clinical Teaching Appointments in Nursing. (1984) King's Fund Report 51, London.

Keane, C.B. (1981) *Management Essentials in Nursing.* Reston Publishing Co. Virginia.

Lathlean, J. & Corner, J. (eds) (1991) *Becoming a Staff Nurse: A guide to the role of the new registered nurse.* Prentice-Hall, London.

Pearson, A. & Vaughan, B. (1986) *Nursing Models for Practice.* Heinemann, London.

Redfern, S.J. (1981) *Hospital Sisters.* Royal College of Nursing, London.

Vaughan, B. & Pillmoor, M. (eds) (1989) *Managing Nursing Work*, Scutari, London.

Walton, M. (1984) *Management and Managing – A Dynamic Approach.* Harper and Row, London.

The Ward Sister's Survival Guide. A collection of articles published in *The Professional Nurse* (1990). Austen Cornish, London.

Chapter 2
Communication

Effective communication is vital for the efficient management of any ward, as outlined in Chapter 1. The purpose of this chapter is to serve as an introduction to some basic communication skills and concepts and to provide some 'food for thought' exercises for those who are interested. There is a Recommended Reading list at the end of the chapter for anyone requiring more detailed information than we have been able to provide.

'Communication' is a difficult word to define. It is apparent to everyone that it is one of life's most basic skills, and yet it is not so simple to achieve it successfully. Kron (1987) defines it as 'the ability to convey ideas and meaning to another person'. Communication implies not just that information has been transmitted from one source, but also that it has been received (in some shape or form) by another. 'Effective communication' implies that the message received is the one that was intended. Effective communication is important in every aspect of patient care and ward management from direct personal interaction with a patient to liaising with the linen room.

Forms of communication

There is often a choice to be made between the methods of communication, though usually more than one type is used at a time. The choice is between:

(1) Verbal communication
(2) Written communication
(3) Non-verbal communication
(4) Symbolic communication.

Verbal communication is the passage of words with a purpose, and is a two-way process. It can be formal or informal, via direct contact or indirectly, by the use of the telephone, for example. It is not a particularly efficient method of communicating because of the many distortions that can arise.

Written communication may be the easiest way of ensuring that a number of people are informed about something, but it has the drawback that it does not offer the reader the opportunity to contribute; there is no interactive communication. The sender of the missive has no means of knowing whether the information has been received as intended, other than by checking later. Written communication is therefore better suited to some messages than to others, and is a useful adjunct to verbal communication.

Non-verbal communication is that which is communicated apart from the verbal message. Non-verbal cues and behaviour include:

- facial expressions and physical appearance
- touch
- postures and gestures
- proximity and positioning
- gaze direction and eye contact
- non-verbal speech such as the use of pauses and 'grunts'.

Most of these have to be seen to be appreciated, but consider also the importance of the tone of voice and the use of non-verbal speech (i.e. 'grunts' etc.) when using the telephone.

Symbolic communication is the message which is sent (consciously or unconsciously) by the symbols chosen by individuals to portray a particular image. These symbols include the badges worn, the choice of hairstyle, the use, or non-use, of make-up, the way the clothes are worn etc.

All these forms of communication can interplay in a single interaction. Often information conveyed by verbal communication can be validated by the accompanying non-verbal communication and supported by written information. This cumulative picture enables the best possible understanding of the message being sent. There are, however, a number of difficulties inherent in communicating effectively. By considering some of them it may be possible to become more aware of the effect they have and so focus on improving skills accordingly. Most of the difficulties we discuss relate to verbal communication, but they are equally applicable to written communication. Little attention is paid here to the complex subject of non-verbal and symbolic communication, but the interested reader should find suitable sources in the Recommended Reading list.

Barriers to effective communication

The sequence of communication consists of the sender putting together a package of information, transmitting it, and then it reaches the receiver and is interpreted. There are three possible areas where distortion of the message can occur. First, the package of information may not accurately reflect the message to be given. Some people are intrinsically better than others at putting their thoughts into words, even in a stress-free environment. The amount of medical and technical terminology and the common use of abbreviations and jargon can make the communication of information even more difficult. It is important to be sure that the terminology and abbreviations are used correctly and that they can be understood by the person receiving the message. Messages should be kept as simple and as clear as possible. It is worth considering written support to verbal communication to ensure that the correct message is sustained.

Second, there may be a problem in the transmission or receipt of the message. The problem may be as basic as an unfamiliar accent, a speech impediment or too soft a voice. There may be a great deal of background noise, or an emotional barrier preventing the recipient from even hearing the words. Finding the 'right' time to pass on a message may be difficult; equally it may be made difficult if the recipient does not want to hear it!

Third, the message may not be interpreted correctly. The correct interpretation of the message depends on a vast number of factors, such as the language used, the timing of the message, the emotive content of the message, the complexity of the information, and whether or not the verbal message agrees with or conflicts with the non-verbal communication. Whether or not the message is expected and the recipient's past experiences all have bearing on the ability to interpret the message correctly.

Another barrier to good communication is lack of sufficient time, or frequent interruptions during communication. Effective communication is aided by frequent checking that the correct message is being received. This is done verbally as well as by checking the non-verbal cues, and is one of the reasons why communication is considered to be a two-way process. If the communication is rushed, incomplete or left without a final check that the message is correct, then it will be less effective.

Communication then is a complex business fraught with potential problems. For the nurse, it is not just a problem of transmitting messages and ensuring that they are correctly received. Communication is also about receiving messages from a variety of sources including patients and other health care workers. Nurses' communication skills are affected by their abilities to initiate, listen, assess, understand and interpret the messages they receive, and by the people who send them.

Communication patterns in the ward and beyond

So far, this chapter has discussed communication as a one-to-one activity, simply for the transmission of information from one individual to another. But within a hospital, there is certain information which needs to be disseminated to, or received from, a wide variety of individuals or groups. Within a ward, the ward sister or charge nurse is often the key figure for the dissemination of information, both into the ward and out of it. There are often patterns or structures in the way in which information is transmitted. These may be formally set up within the formal organization, or informal within the ward group. The important thing is that the communication must be effective. Different patterns of communication may be more or less effective, and normally a range of the patterns is used to cover all the types of information and responsibilities. Some examples of different communication networks are given, together with some of their advantages and disadvantages.

The Wheel Network

With a radial communication system there is someone at the centre of the circle coordinating things. The dotted lines in Figure 2.1 represent the possible informal communication patterns. This system can be most effective and provides every opportunity for two-way communication. The sister or charge nurse receives feedback from the nursing team, taking in and feeding out communications and coordinating the whole. In this way everyone has an opportunity to feel involved. If working properly, the Wheel Network means that communication is faster, fewer errors are made and fewer messages are needed. The nurse at the centre of the wheel does not need to be the ward sister or charge nurse. When considering direct patient care this person might be the patient's primary nurse.

The ward sister or charge nurse does not necessarily have to communicate with all groups, for if the nursing team is organized and supervised more of the information can be directed through the team members. It is important, however, that the sister or charge nurse keeps in touch with what is going on. This information can be obtained at the daily ward report when feedback is received from the nursing team.

Within the ward, interaction occurs between various groups, for example, doctors with patients and social workers with patients'

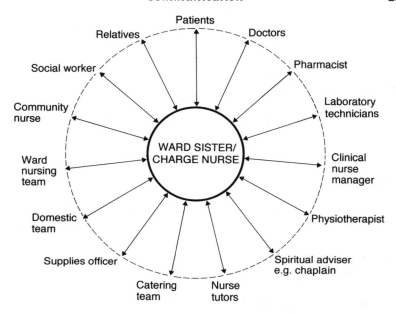

Fig. 2.1 The Wheel Network.

relatives. The person at the centre of the wheel must keep in touch with what is happening and be aware of what information has been given to patients or their relatives, what investigations are arranged and any plans made for discharge. These must all be documented (Fig. 2.2).

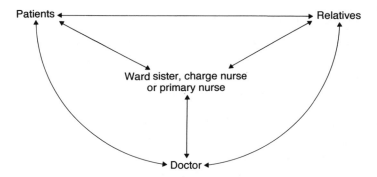

Fig. 2.2 Interaction between ward sister/charge nurse or primary nurse and patients, doctors and patients' relatives.

The Chain Network

An alternative to the 'wheel' of communication, is the 'chain' of communication where the information goes in a line from top to bottom. Within the nursing team, all communication originates with the nurse in charge and is passed down the line. There is little opportunity for feedback and a feeling is created amongst the nurses that their contribution is worthless. The formal pattern of communication set by an organisation is often a chain network.

Open communication

An open communication network, where every nurse is able to communicate with everyone else, can be valuable when an important issue is to be decided and a variety of views are sought. It can be very time-consuming, but if all the staff are to feel involved or the issue is complex, then it should be considered. It is not suitable for everyday use as it can become very confused.

Sociologists have looked at the way in which work is managed in hospitals, not only by nurses, but by all the various health professionals. Strauss (1971; 1979) developed a theory in which the hospital is a place where all personnel are involved in complex negotiations in order to achieve their personal and professional objectives as well as those of the institution. The communication patterns and relationships between individuals reflect their position in this 'negotiated order'. The extent to which the ward sister or charge nurse is successful in reaching negotiated outcomes reflects their position in this 'negotiated order'. It is a function of their professional status and current job grading as well as the impact they have as a manager.

Relationships and their effects on communication

The relationships between all the members of the health care team have considerable effect on, and are affected by, the communication skills of the sister or charge nurse. Since the ward sister or charge nurse is the key figure in the ward communication network (Lelean, 1973), her attitudes to the other members of the team have an impact on the ability of the whole team to communicate effectively.

The status hierarchy of the group may affect the flow of communication. Status is the position an individual holds within a group and is usually assessed in terms of the degree of responsibility which that person carries. Status can either be formal – given by the formal organization as is the case of the ward sister or charge nurse – or it can be informal – given by the group. If the sister or charge nurse has both formal and informal status this will be good for the morale of the ward and the communication network should be good. Informal status depends on several factors: the personality of the individual, the degree of contribution made to the group, her or his degree of knowledge, ability, skill and generosity.

Because of a status higher than that of the rest of the group, the ward sister or charge nurse must take the lead, realizing that because of this status subordinates may find communication difficult. In order to overcome this, every effort must be made to create a feeling of importance in all the nurses. This can be achieved by:

- Direct communication between the sister or charge nurse and *all* grades of nurse within the team
- Making sure they know what is expected of them
- Giving them a sense of responsibility, and a share in making decisions.

Some nurses consider doctors to be of a higher status than themselves. The nursing team and medical team, however, each have their own role and are complementary to each other in the care of the patients. If nurses lack confidence and are unsure of themselves they may find communication with the doctor difficult and this may lead to misunderstanding and communication breakdown. Some doctors think they have a right to state what nursing care is needed by a patient. This is, however, a nursing responsibility although in some instances discussion with the doctor may be indicated.

The sister or charge nurse has a responsibility to make the members of the nursing team aware of their distinct role in patient care. Planning care and proper planned discharge of patients are two aspects of this special role. If she or he is seen to make a firm stand, insisting that the nurses decide on the nursing care required or that patients are not discharged until suitable arrangements can be made, they will follow this example and act likewise. Status can also affect the communication between nurse and doctor, depending on their positions in their respective hierarchies and whether they consider this to be important or not. The sister or charge nurse may be able to communicate with the consultants more effectively than other nurses, partly because of their status, but also because they have often worked with each other for some time and have developed respect for each other's views and skills. A less experienced nurse may not be so well known to the doctor, so her skills may not be appreciated or her views accepted as a consequence. Of course this will depend on the approachability of those concerned, their temperaments and personalities, and also on the importance of what is being communicated.

Different personality traits affect communication and can be instrumental in its breakdown. A nurse with a dominant personality often has difficulty in fitting in with other members of the group and may also show aggressiveness towards colleagues. This attitude will build up a barrier and inhibit communication.

If a newly appointed sister or charge nurse lacks confidence she or he may give the impression of being a bossy person, giving orders but never asking. This will cause resentment and uncertainty throughout the ward team, including nursing, domestic and clerical staff. This resentment will inhibit communication between them and the sister or charge nurse, and in some instances between the different groups of staff within the ward, for example nurses and domestics. This approach also has an inhibiting effect on patients and relatives.

Effects of breakdown in communication

If the communication network breaks down, it can lead to serious problems which often result in an inefficiently run ward. In many instances, distress to patients will occur and there may be cause for official complaints to be made against the hospital. If all staff are not aware of 'what is going on', they become unhappy and unsettled, their morale becomes low and this results in a breakdown of communication between staff, patients and their relatives.

Where communication is ineffective within the nursing team there will be insecurity, a lack of job satisfaction and little motivation. If too little time is spent communicating with the groups which make up the nursing team such as day and night staff, a lack of understanding of one another's problems may develop which will result in each group blaming the other for mistakes or omissions which occur. This will lead to hostility between the groups, although their aims and objectives are the same. Hostility may also occur between different day shifts for the same reason.

In a ward where importance is not attached to communication, matters of consequence are neglected. Fluid balance charts and observation charts are not completed accurately, and important aspects of nursing care are overlooked. Explanations to patients and relatives tend to be omitted or these people may be misinformed.

If the patients are given inadequate information on admission to the ward such as ward routine, the significance of the different uniforms or the probable length of stay in hospital, they may experience difficulty in adapting to hospital. If, once in the ward, they receive conflicting information regarding progress, operation date, preparation for operation, information relating to special procedures, probable discharge date and so forth, patients and their relatives will become unhappy, annoyed and even hostile. This will lead to a strained relationship between the patients and the ward nurses.

When ineffective communication exists between departments within the hospital, conflict arises. There is also a lack of understanding of each other's objectives and problems. Staff in other departments may become uncooperative and this will eventually have a detrimental effect on patient care.

The 'ward report' or 'handover'

Time must be set aside on a regular basis so the nurses are given the opportunity to communicate with each other, both verbally and in writing. It is of paramount importance that nurses are given time to think and communicate in the same way as doctors. This may prove difficult at times but nurse-to-nurse communication must be rated as a high priority, and recognized by all as a vital part of the nurses' day.

In order that those present can concentrate on receiving and giving information, a quiet place on the ward should be used, away from the ward activity, visitors and *all* telephones. The most suitable place will depend on the facilities available on that particular ward; this could be the patients' dayroom, the ward office, or the bathroom or linen room in a less-modern ward. Attempting to hold a ward report in the Nurses' Station can be like trying to hold a session in the middle of Heathrow airport!

The time set aside can be referred to as the *handover* or the *daily ward report*. This is a two-way process, enabling the sister or charge nurse to obtain essential feedback from the nurses delivering the bedside care. It is possible to set a certain time aside on a regular basis despite the pressures of the ward, if each member of the ward team accepts that proper communication is vital for the efficient running of the ward. The pattern, once set, should be adhered to even when the going is tough, although it may be adapted to a particular situation, depending on the time available. It should be emphasized that the busier the ward, the greater the need for spending time on passing on relevant information to *all* members.

There are a great number of reasons why the ward report is carried out; some of them are overt and purposeful, as shown below, but in addition it has the great benefit of providing a forum for staff support and allows the ward sister or charge nurse an opportunity to define the ward atmosphere. The purposes for the ward report include:

(1) Discussion of current state of the patients in the ward, including their nursing needs
(2) Problem-solving specific patient problems
(3) Evaluating nursing action and discussion of rationale for pre-scribed care
(4) Communication about pending admissions, bed state etc.
(5) Forum for the airing of anxieties, problems or issues related to patient care or other professional matters
(6) Feedback for the person in charge about what activity has taken place and what remains to be done
(7) Opportunity for identifying and fulfilling (in part) nurses' educational needs.

During the daily ward report, most ward nursing staff should be present so that each nurse is given the opportunity to keep herself or himself fully informed. When discussing patients all the nurses must bear in mind that there will be some nurses present who have returned from holiday or days-off, and they must indicate an awareness of the importance of emphasizing what has occurred in their absence. Guidance from the sister or charge nurse may be necessary.

The times and methods of communication sessions and handover reports will vary according to the needs of the nursing team on each ward and department. Indeed, it may change from day to day to accommodate different purposes for the report. One day may be designated as a teaching report session, during which patients' medical diagnosis or nursing problems are discussed and explained in detail. Another day's report session may be designed to include a social worker, or other health care worker who can update the nursing team on any issues involving the ward patients or other ward-related issues. On the days when special report sessions take place, it may be possible to have a brief handover first, to ensure that information about the patients is passed on to all nurses.

Recent studies into nurses' working patterns (Ball *et al*, 1989) indicate that ward reports and handovers are one of the biggest consumers of nursing time. Usually only minimal and essential nursing care takes place at the time of the report, as all or most of the nurses are involved in the report session. If the report takes an hour, and eight or ten nurses are involved, this time represents a whole day's work for one nurse. It is small wonder that managers are looking at the reporting sessions and questioning their worth. It is therefore very important to ensure that reports are managed in the best possible way, with minimal time-wasting and gossiping, and as little repetition as possible. After all, written communication, in the form of patient care plans, should serve as the prime method of communicating patient care, and the ward report should be seen as a supplement. The day-to-day running of the ward does not only involve direct patient care, and the value of the ward report session for the discussion and communication of other issues should ensure that it continues to have an important place in the daily routine.

'Walk round' reports, with discussion at the patient's bedside, are becoming more acceptable to both patients and nurses. An opportunity is given for the patients to be involved in decisions about their care with a chance to talk about needs and problems which have been identified by the patient or the nurses. This type of report may be suitable for all the reporting sessions throughout the day, or can be used in conjunction with the in-depth 'sit down' handovers, e.g. 'walk round' reports at the changeover between day and night staff and an in-depth handover during the day.

Ward meetings

As the ward nursing team covers a 24-hour period it is often difficult to ensure that all the nurses are kept informed of issues relating to the directorate, the hospital or the health district. Staff must be made aware of such things as changes in policies and procedures, and information from meetings such as the health and safety at work committee and unit meetings.

Regular ward meetings to discuss these matters are invaluable and it is an advantage if a member of the night nursing team can attend but this is not always possible. An opportunity for a ward meeting could be at lunch-time or during the afternoon overlap. Ideally the ward meetings should follow the sisters' and charge nurses' unit meeting. The meetings will provide a time for the ward staff to discuss matters relating to the ward such as clinical, managerial and personnel topics. If an opportunity is given to the staff to talk over problems other than those related directly to patient care, and to discuss proposed changes within the ward, a breakdown in communication amongst members of the ward team should be minimized. This will also be aided by including members of the night nursing team. Notes of the meeting could be taken for the benefit of those unable to attend.

Regular peer group meetings for student nurses can be very beneficial, giving them an opportunity to talk objectively about their allocation to the ward, highlighting the negative as well as the positive aspects. If taken as constructive criticism and acted upon, patient care and student teaching should be enhanced. The ward sister or charge nurse will need to be called at the end of the meeting so that the various issues can be brought to her or his attention, and any explanation given if indicated. The points raised can then be discussed at the next ward meeting.

Bulletin board

A bulletin board such as a small notice board, situated in an area accessible to and used by all the nurses, can be used for displaying information which needs to be conveyed to all members of the ward team. It must, however, be kept up-to-date otherwise the staff will take little notice of it. Alternatively, a communications book, available to all staff could be used for the same purpose. These aids should supplement ward meetings but never replace them, and are a useful way of dealing with the many memos and circulars received.

Unit meetings

Most clinical nurse managers hold regular meetings with the sisters and charge nurses in the unit in an attempt to keep everyone informed of activities and changes within the unit, the hospital and the health district. These meetings must be a two-way process as the clinical nurse manager requires feedback from the sisters and charge nurses. This gives the sisters and charge nurses an opportunity to put forward ideas and suggestions to enhance patient care as well as to discuss any day-to-day problems.There needs to be, however, a sense of trust between the clinical nurse manager and sisters and charge nurses so that ideas can be freely exchanged.

Written nursing communication

It has been the practice for nurses to write as briefly as possible in the nursing report, with 'good day', 'good night', 'no change' and so forth. It has sometimes been suggested that with long-term patients within an acute ward, there is no need to make a daily entry about the patient. However, written communication is essential today as there is a continuing team of nurses concerned with patient care, with many more nurses involved in the patient's care over a period of time, for example, stoma nurse, mastectomy nurse specialist, community nurse, ward nurses. There are more part-time nurses, including agency and 'bank' nurses; often a quicker turnover of nursing staff; the working week is shorter; more doctors are involved in any one patient's care and the patients are discharged more quickly.

As communication is at risk everything relating to each patient must be well documented, so that all nurses are aware of what has been done and what is to be done for each patient. Every nurse needs to be aware of the patient's background, so that his or her needs will be known when plans are being made for his or her care and discharge home. It is no longer enough that this sort of information is retained by the ward sister or charge nurse and not fully documented – it must be available to the nursing team. For example, a patient who has had a cerebrovascular accident and who lives in a house with steep narrow stairs and an outside toilet, will need arrangements made to have a bed brought downstairs and a commode obtained. Efficient and adequate documentation leads to good communication and aids the delivery and continuity of a high standard of care.

Systems of recording are many, and include records for individual hospitals, nursing information sheets, nursing history sheets, nursing care plans, work books and report books. If everything relating to the patient is included in the nursing records, avoiding the need for work books and work lists, which detract from an individualized approach to patient care, greater efficiency should result. In most hospitals the nursing process approach to care is used, with the associated nursing history and assessment, care plan and written evaluation.

The overall aim of the nursing records is to chart the progress of the patient, and any changes relating to the patient's physical or psychological care during the period in hospital, and to communicate the changes and progress to all members of the nursing team. The way the nursing record is organized will reflect the model of nursing care used in the ward. The information recorded must be accurate and factual (the facts being objective and not subjective), and needs to include changes in mobility, mental state, progress to independence and dietary and fluid intake. Other points need to be included, such as sleep patterns, abnormal signs and symptoms, observations, accidents and untoward incidents. Information given to the doctor must be noted, and also the action taken. It is always advisable to include the doctor's name. The state of wounds and removal of drains, clips or sutures, and details of the preparation for tests and operations, followed by post treatment or postoperative details, must be fully recorded. Changes in nursing care and medical and surgical treatment, and the action taken are also entered in the nursing record.

Any information given to the patient or relatives by either the nurse or doctor is recorded and whether the patient or relatives are aware of his or her diagnosis and prognosis. These both need to be continually updated. Relevant information given to the nurse by patients or their relatives is also recorded. Complaints made by patients or relatives are recorded in detail in the records of the patient concerned (see Chapter 12).

Each entry in the nursing record must be clearly written, dated, timed and signed. It cannot be overemphasized that the nursing record is a legal document and may need to be referred back to in the event of a query or complaint, therefore nothing should be omitted. This is becoming increasingly important as more people are becoming litigation-minded (see Chapter 12).

The use of abbreviations is dangerous since it can alter or confuse the meaning of what is being said and may have far reaching implications, resulting in delays or even errors.

As the management of hospitals becomes more and more business-like, ward sisters and charge nurses will be expected to write reports for meetings and to attend and contribute to management meetings. Their ability to write well, to put over an argument and back it up with facts and figures, may be important to their control over change within the ward. Nurses who have charge of wards or units will have to become expert, not only in writing, but also in reading (and reading between the lines!) the reports that such a business-style management produces. More information about analysing and presenting data can be found in Chapter 4.

Summary

This chapter has looked at the subject of communication and has attempted to provide some basic concepts relating to the topic. It has looked at some of the forms of communication and some of the barriers to communication in general. Communication patterns within health care settings and the relationships between the various members of the health care team all have an impact on the ability of the leader of the ward to ensure good communication and effective management. The importance of good written communication has been highlighted but little guidance as to how to develop good writing skills has been provided. References for further information are provided at the end of the chapter.

This chapter has focused on communication within the ward, in general, and between the members of the multidisciplinary team. Communicating with patients and their families is just as vital to their wellbeing, and is more fully discussed in Chapters 6, 7 and 8, with emphasis made on the dying patient and family in Chapter 9.

Topics for discussion

1. Forms of communication:

> Mr Maple was being starved for clinical investigation. Unfortunately he was rather vague and was given a cup of tea by a nurse. Mr Maple was kept in hospital much longer than necessary as the investigation had to be postponed until the next available appointment, which was three days later.

Discuss the possible reasons for this communication breakdown, identifying verbal, written and non-verbal cues that should or could have been identified and prevented the occurrence.

2. The effects of poor communication:

> Mrs Oak lived alone and arrangements were made for her discharge from hospital, but no one informed her relatives as each member of the team thought that someone else was doing it. Mrs Oak was taken home by ambulance to find that she was unable to get into her flat as her niece had got the key. Furthermore, the flat was cold and there was no food for her. Her relatives made an official complaint to the hospital.

Discuss reasons how and why such an omission by the nursing staff might have happened, and make suggestions, for inclusion in a report to your manager, as to how such an omission might be prevented in the future.

3. Make list of non-verbal cues and behaviour and try to identify each of them and their meaning in their particular context, in interactions you observe at work. Suggestions:

- Use of eye contact
- Posture, including arm position – folded or open
- Body contact and positioning
- Telephone technique
- 'Hidden meaning'.

References

Ball, J.A., Hurst, K., Booth, M.R. and Franklin, R. (1989) *But who will make the beds? – A research based strategy for ward nursing skills and resources for the 1990s* The report of the Mersey region project on assessment of nurse staffing and support worker requirements for acute general hospitals, Nuffield Institute of Health Service Studies and Mersey Regional Health Authority.

Catterton, J. (1988) How busy are you? ... Ward Activity *Nursing Times*, Nov 9, 15. **84**(45).

Kron, T. (1987) *The Management of Nursing Care – putting leadership skills to work* (6th ed.), Saunders Co., Philadelphia.

Strauss, A. (1979) *Negotiations: Varieties, Contexts, Processes and Social Order*, Josey-Bass Publishers.

Strauss, A. *et al.* (1971) The Hospital and its Negotiated Order in Castles, F.G. (ed.) *Decisions, Organizations and Society*, Penguin Books.

Recommended Reading

Altschul, A.T. (1972) *Patient–Nurse Interaction* Churchill-Livingstone, Edinburgh.

Bridge, W. & Macleod Clarke, J. (ed.) *Communication in Nursing Care.* Education for Care Series H.M. & Publishers, Aylesbury.

Burnard, P. (1989) *Effective communication skills for health professionals*, Chapman and Hall, London.

Faulkner, A. (ed) (1984) *Communication. Recent Advances in Nursing.* Churchill-Livingstone, Edinburgh.

Fletcher, J. (1983) *How to Write a Report.* Institute of Personnel Management, London.

Hayward, J. (1975) *Information – a Prescription Against Pain.* Royal College of Nursing, London.

Horne, E.M. (ed.) (1990) *Effective Communication*, Austen Cornish, London.

King's Fund Project Paper 21 (1979) *A Handbook for Nurse-to-Nurse Reporting.*

Lelean, S.R. (1973) *Ready for Report, Nurse?*, Royal College of Nursing, London.

Salvage, J. (1988) How to be assertive. *Nursing Standard* **2**, July 9, p 19.

Walton, M. (1984) *Management and Managing – A Dynamic Approach.* Harper and Row, London.

Chapter 3
Taking on a new ward

Taking on a new ward is a big step, especially when it is the first post as a sister or charge nurse. On moving from one ward or hospital to another, it is likely that the person will have a mental check list of those things to be noted in a new situation, but the newly-appointed sister or charge nurse may find a guide useful.

All new staff should have an orientation plan developed to meet their individual needs. For a new sister or charge nurse the development of this plan will be the responsibility of the clinical nurse manager or professional development nurse and should be done in conjunction with the new appointee to ensure that individual needs and areas of interest are covered. The orientation programme will provide written and verbal information about a variety of topics, some of which will include:

- Standards expected
- Philosophy of the hospital
- Layout of the hospital with list of wards, ward sisters and consultants
- Location of departments plus introduction to heads of departments
- Demonstration of emergency procedures
- Admission and discharge procedures
- Appraisal system
- Confidential information policy
- Communication patterns
- Legal implications of nurses' actions
- The extended role of the nurse
- Nursing policies and procedures
- Operational policies
- Relationship within the nursing structure
- Lines of accountability
- College of nursing and link tutor
- Budgets
- Relationship with community nursing service
- Facilities for ward sisters, including changing facilities.

Those hospitals that hold or are working towards trust status will probably place greater emphasis on business plans and mission statements, quality assurance measures and facts and figures. Whatever it includes, the information gathered during the orientation period will form a foundation on which to build once in the ward. In an ideal situation the orientation will take place over a period of time.

Once in the ward, the process of collecting information must continue. The sister's orientation to the ward can be categorized as:

- Familiarization with those persons having a direct or indirect contribution to patient care
- Information exclusive to the ward
- Information exclusive to the hospital
- Information exclusive to the health authority

Familiarization with personnel

The Management Structure

In 1983 an enquiry into the management of the National Health Service recommended a need for more effective management, with close financial control and speedier decision-making at every level of the Service. Changes in management were suggested, the aim being to improve the quality of the service given to the patient and to enhance the level of support received by those giving direct patient care, making the Service more cost-effective. The report is known as the Griffiths Report.

The White Paper, 'Working for Patients' (1989), aims at reforming further the National Health Service, giving hospital staff more control in running their own affairs, improving efficiency, making the quality of the Service more explicit, giving patients a greater choice and staff greater job satisfaction. Hospitals can either be directly managed by a Health Authority or be self-governing, i.e. NHS Trusts – the latter is the model for the future. NHS Trusts are directly accountable to the NHS Management Executive and are managed by a Trust Board, comprising a chairman, chief executive, executive (including a director of nursing) and non-executive members. (See Fig 3.1.)

The role of all hospitals, however, will be similar – to provide services through previously agreed contracts with 'purchasers', e.g. District Health Authorities, general medical practices having their own budget, private hospitals.

Contracts will ensure that the 'purchasers', who buy services accord-

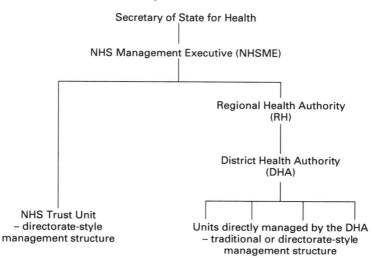

Fig. 3.1 Management accountability of NHS Trusts and Directly Managed Units within the NHS.

ing to the needs of the population they serve, will receive an agreed level of service at an agreed quality and cost. Hospital Trusts are directly accountable to the Secretary of State for Health, they have full control over their own finances and are able to take initiatives in order to improve care and services for their patients.

Management arrangements are being restructured in different ways in both trust and directly managed hospitals. These structures are varied ranging from the 'traditional style' to directorate models. Directorates may be clinical, e.g. medical, surgical, or non-clinical, e.g. radiology. The head of each directorate has an obligation to ensure that unit policy is carried out and undertakes day-to-day management within the directorate, being responsible to the trust or unit management board for control of the budget. Each directorate has a management team comprising a consultant, senior nurse, business manager and financial adviser. Devolution of resources enables each directorate to make decisions and take initiatives closer to where care is given involving care staff in the process. Whatever style of hospital management is employed, the personnel with whom the ward sister or charge nurse works will be the same.

The personnel can be subdivided as:

(1) Nursing
(2) Medical

(3)   Other ward members
(4)   Other health care workers
(5)   Others – non-specific
(6)   Heads of departments.

Nursing personnel

The nursing team, if interpreted on a broad basis, consists of:

- Ward nursing team
- Nursing management
- Nursing education
- Community nursing service
- Specialist Nurses.

Ward nursing team

The team will include qualified nurses, student nurses, support workers and auxiliary nurses. In many hospitals it may include a second ward sister or charge nurse.

The sister or charge nurse must get to know the ward staff as soon as possible, gaining their confidence and recognizing their capabilities and potential. It is important to acknowledge that everyone has a valuable contribution to make.

To help to achieve this, it is essential to make an effort to introduce oneself to each team member as soon as possible. This will encourage them to feel more at ease and less threatened. It should be noted that as a 24-hour service is given it may be several days before all team members are met.

Job descriptions should be available for each nurse member of the team and it will be necessary to become familiar with these as soon as possible.

Qualified nurses

The roles of first- and second-level nurses are not interchangeable because they each follow different training programmes. First-level nurses are registered nurses, enrolled nurses are second-level nurses. Although the position of the enrolled nurse is safeguarded with the advent of Project 2000 (see Chapter 11), enrolled nurses are being actively encouraged to convert to first-level nurses. Recent changes at the UKCC allow enrolled and registered nurses to entitle themselves 'Registered nurse'. The grading will encompass their roles and responsibilities rather than specific training received. However, for guidance regarding the capabilities of newly qualified registered or enrolled nurses, the competencies for which each are prepared are detailed below.

Registered Nurse or First-Level Nurse:

(1) Advise on the promotion of health and the prevention of illness.
(2) Recognize situations that may be detrimental to the health and well-being of the individual.
(3) Carry out those activities involved when conducting the comprehensive assessment of a person's nursing requirements.
(4) Recognize the significance of the observations made, and use these to develop an initial nursing assessment.
(5) Devise a plan of nursing care based on the assessment, with the co-operation of the patient, to the extent that this is possible, taking into account the medical prescription.
(6) Implement the planned programme of nursing care, and where appropriate teach and co-ordinate other members of the caring team who may be responsible for implementing specific aspects of the nursing care.
(7) Review the effectiveness of the nursing case provided, and where appropriate, initiate any action that may be required.
(8) Work in a team with other nurses, and with medical and paramedical staff and social workers.
(9) Undertake the management of the care of a group of patients over a period of time and organize the appropriate support services related to the care of the particular type of patient with whom she is likely to come in contact.

The registered nurse is also responsible for her ongoing, personal and professional development.

Enrolled Nurse or Second-Level Nurse

The second-level nurse works under the direction of a registered nurse and is able to:

(1) Assist in carrying out comprehensive observation of the patient and help in assessing her or his care requirements.
(2) Develop skills to enable her or him to assist in the implementation of nursing care under the direction of a Registered General Nurse, Registered Mental Nurse, Registered Nurse for the Mentally Handicapped or Registered Sick Children's Nurse.

(3)   Accept delegated nursing tasks.
(4)   Assist in reviewing the effectiveness of the care provided.
(5)   Work in a team with other nurses, and with medical and para-
      medical staff and social workers.

It will be helpful to find out what the support workers and nursing
auxiliaries are taught during their in-service training. In the case of
student nurses, the stage of training they have reached, previous
experience gained, and what experience they can expect to gain whilst
in the ward will be valuable information to the new sister or charge
nurse.

It must be remembered that the senior staff nurse has probably been in
charge of the ward whilst awaiting the appointment of a new sister or
charge nurse and may have gained informal status and be looked upon
as the leader in that ward. With the arrival of the newly appointed person
the staff nurse may feel threatened and appear resentful and aggressive.
The new sister or charge nurse can help by being kind and understanding, and ensuring that the staff nurse understands that she or he is
depending on the staff nurse's help and support.

It is disastrous to immediately force ideas and views upon the
established ward staff. The putting forward of alternative methods and
ideas must wait until a firm relationship has been built up and this will
take time. The sister or charge nurse should be accepted by the team if
the guidelines laid down in Chapter 1 are followed.

Nursing management structure

As the interpretation of the Griffiths management structures and recent
management initiatives vary from hospital to hospital, it is not possible
to describe in detail the nursing management structure. It is, therefore,
imperative that newly appointed ward sisters and charge nurses ensure
that they are aware to whom they are accountable for both managerial
and professional matters within their hospital or unit, as there are
several models of management. Regardless of the local model it is a
requirement that every Trust Board has an executive director of nursing,
who will provide professional advice to the board, as well as carrying out
other functions.

Nursing education structure

Nurse education is undertaken in colleges of nursing and midwifery in
partnership with service areas. Colleges often cover several Health

Authorities/Trusts/Units and there is usually a locally based education centre within a hospital. There is close collaboration between the college, the appropriate National Board and an Institute of Higher Education. On successful completion of the training or qualifying course the nurse will have a nursing qualification and in addition a diploma or a degree awarded. In some instances the independent sector may also be involved in providing training areas of specialist input.

The management structure of each college of nursing will vary (see Fig. 3.2) but each will have a principal or dean supported by vice-principals or assistant principals, each with different areas of responsibility. The dean or principal is equivalent to a chief executive managing pre- and post-registration nurse education within the area covered by the college.

Firm links are formed between the college and each ward and department involved in nurse education. The sister or charge nurse needs to make sure she or he knows the education and clinical link persons for her or his ward. The link persons will endeavour to ensure that all members of the ward team are kept up-to-date with changes in the college as they occur.

Joint appointments between nursing service and nursing education are being introduced into some nursing education structures (see Chapter 1).

As structures will vary from one authority to another it is not possible to illustrate the structure specifically, but an example is shown in Fig. 3.2.

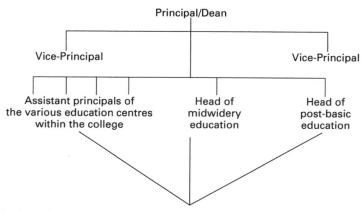

Registered nurse tutors, specialist nurses, lecturers, lecturer/practitioners (may have links with a specified clinical area or group of students depending on their area of interest or academic qualification)

Fig. 3.2 One example of a nurse education structure.

Community nursing service

This includes district nurses, school nurses, midwives and health visitors. The involvement of these nurses at ward level will depend on the local policy. The district nurse and health visitor may visit the ward on a regular basis. On the other hand, there may be a liaison district nursing sister based in the hospital who acts as a link between hospital and community, being available to visit the patients whilst they are in hospital and then referring them to the appropriate nurse in the community. It is very important to know the lines of communication which exist in the district so that the community nursing service can always be contacted.

Specialist nurses

Specialist and consultant nurses are developing their role and cover many aspects of nursing. The availability of these nurses with special knowledge will vary from health authority to health authority. It is important to be aware of any service provided and how to make use of it (see Chapter 8).

Medical personnel

The ward may have one consultant attached, or as many as five or six. This will affect the number of doctors the sister or charge nurse will have to get to know as shown in Fig. 3.3.

In a teaching hospital, there will be more doctors attached to a consultant than in a non-teaching hospital, and each consultant will have a responsibility for a number of medical students who will have a clinical involvement in the ward. It will be an advantage to get to know consultants from other wards and specialists to whom patients may be referred.

Other ward members

This group will include some or all of the following:

- Ward clerk or secretary
- Ward assistant
- Ward orderly
- Domestic assistant
- Volunteers – Hospital League of Friends, WRVS, Red Cross.

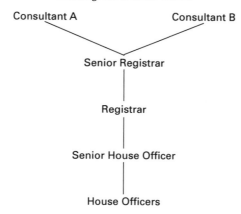

Fig. 3.3 The number of doctors a ward sister/charge nurse of one ward may have to get to know.

It is important to introduce oneself to each one as they come to the ward, getting to know them and gaining their confidence, recognizing their contribution and that they are part of the team and have received appropriate training. It will be necessary to find out the content of their job, the involvement of the sister or charge nurse in the supervision of their work and to whom each is responsible. In some hospitals, certain ancillary staff may be responsible to an outside contractor, and they will probably adhere rigidly to the work schedules agreed when the contract was negotiated.

If contractors are involved, the sister or charge nurse has a responsibility for making sure she or he is aware of the contract, and that it is fulfilled. In the case of volunteers they are usually responsible to the volunteer organizer or unit administrator. The sister or charge nurse, however, has sapiential authority over these members of the ward team. This means that whilst working in the ward they are also responsible to the sister or charge nurse as well as to their line manager for that part of their job which takes place within the ward.

Other health care workers

Health care workers who may be involved at ward level are:

- Social worker
- Physiotherapist
- Speech therapist
- Therapeutic radiographer
- Occupational therapist.

The health care workers' involvement will be determined by the needs of the patient and the type of ward concerned.

The sister or charge nurse will need to know the role of each health care worker, and how referrals are made to them. The roles of each member will be discussed later in the book. Some referrals will be from the nursing staff, others from the doctor and in the case of the social worker the patient may also refer himself. It is important to know how to contact these personnel when needed. Some health care workers may visit the ward on a daily basis making referral much easier.

The sister or charge nurse will also be expected to know how to contact health care workers out of normal working hours in case an emergency arises.

Others

Other hospital personnel who may be involved at ward level are:

- Spiritual adviser
- Dietician
- ECG technician
- Diagnostic radiographer
- Chiropodist
- Appliance officer
- Maintenance engineers
- Laboratory technicians
- Research workers
- Porters.

As with the health care workers, it is necessary to know the role of each of the personnel mentioned, and the method of contacting them during the day and in some instances, such as a patient's spiritual adviser being needed, out of normal hours or in an emergency.

Heads of departments

During orientation to the hospital, the various departments may have been visited and the head of each department met. The departments concerned include:

- Domestic services
- Supplies
- Laundry

- Central sterile supply department
- Catering
- Medical records
- Engineering and maintenance
- Radiography
- ECG
- Social work
- Physiotherapy
- Mortuary
- Pharmacy
- Haematology, bacteriology and pathology.

Most of these departments are a daytime service, Monday to Friday only, but this varies from one hospital to another. In many instances a member of the department will be on call to provide emergency cover, and will be contacted either by the doctor or hospital administrator if required, depending on the hospital policy.

Activities relating to other departments which must be known by the ward staff if the ward is to run smoothly are:

- How and when to order patients' meals
- How to order a special diet
- How to order sterile supplies
- How to order other supplies, including pharmaceuticals
- How to arrange repair of fittings, fixtures and equipment
- Obtaining blood for transfusion and blood derivatives
- How to obtain case notes, X-rays
- The time the departments are open, e.g., Saturday morning
- Action to take if the ward becomes short of linen, drugs, sterile supplies at evenings or weekends
- How to arrange patient transport within the hospital
- How to arrange patient transport for discharge.

Information exclusive to the ward

Certain information will vary from one ward to another and it will be necessary to become familiar with this information. This should include:

- Ward philosophy for care
- Nursing care model used (if any)
- Care plan structure

- Nursing quality initiatives
- Pattern of the patient's day
- Pattern of the nurses' day
- Ward geography – layout, and location of annexes
- Allocation of beds to consultants
- Admission days – list and emergency
- Theatre days
- Consultants' rounds – day and time
- Consultants' clinic days
- Location of emergency equipment
    fire fighting
    resuscitation
    tracheostomy
    oxygen
    suction
- location of, and how to use, special equipment such as
    hoist
    monitor
    defibrillator
    humidifier
    special mattress
    automatic infusion pump
    ventilator
- Any other information specific to the ward.

Information exclusive to the hospital

Information that relates to the hospital as a whole will often be covered during orientation to the hospital, and includes:

- Emergency procedures
    fire
    cardiac arrest
    major disaster
    bomb alert
    radiation hazard
    patient for emergency surgery
    security systems
- Routine ordering of all supplies
    food stores
    patients' meals
    stationery

    linen

    sterile supplies

    appliances

    pharmaceuticals

    new equipment

- Maintenance, routinely and out of hours
- Barrier nursing

    policy

    disposal of infected linen

    cleaning of room following infection

- Disposal of soiled linen
- Portering service
- Laboratory services and collection of specimens
- Admission procedure including how to obtain notes and X-rays
- Visiting arrangements
- Ambulance arrangements
- Discharge procedure including booking appointments, ordering ambulances and contacting the community nursing service
- Discharge against medical advice
- Death of patients
- Transfer of patients between wards and theatre
- Transfer of patients to other wards or hospitals
- Car parking facilities for visitors and staff
- Arrangements for staff to book holidays.

Information exclusive to the health authority

Information which relates to the district is based on nursing procedures and nursing policies.

Nursing procedures

The procedures are usually found in a nursing procedure manual, which is standard for wards and departments within a hospital. A nursing procedure is an established and uniform method of performing nursing activity, and gives specific information for those performing the procedure. Alternatively, procedures may be based on principles rather than specific details. Procedures should not be so rigid that any changes are discouraged, and regular review is therefore essential. A copy of the procedure manual is usually available in each ward and department.

    Procedure manuals are now being written from a research base and the reasons for each step of the procedure are fully explained.

Nursing policy

Nursing policy is a way of ensuring that the philosophy and goals for the nursing service are applied uniformly throughout the organisation, forming a framework within which everyone works. Policies act as a guide for the nurse managers when making decisions but, most important, they safeguard both patient and nurse. A nursing policy manual is found in each ward and department in most hospitals. Nursing policy should originate with those who are doing the job, although it is finally agreed at senior level. The sister or charge nurse has a responsibility to become familiar with the nursing policies, making a special note of such issues as:

- Control of drug stocks at ward level
- Medical students undertaking locums
- Prescribing drugs and implication of accepting verbal prescriptions
- Complaints procedure for patients and relatives
- Grievance procedure for staff
- Disciplinary procedure
- Accident procedure for patients, visitors, staff
- Gratuities, wills, gifts
- Private and amenity patients
- Management of violent patients and the use of restraints
- Types of leave available for nurses
- Occupational health service
- Provision of information to press and police
- Policy relating to research
- Nursing care of female patients by male nurses
- Adoption of new equipment
- Allocation of student nurses to wards and departments.

Summary

The taking on of a new ward is an exciting time for the newly appointed sister or charge nurse. There is a lot to learn and a lot to achieve. This chapter has attempted to provide a few guidelines as a framework for identifying the people and things that need to be met and discovered quickly to enable the rapid orientation to the ward. A full and unhurried orientation may allow the individual to settle into the new role more easily. Only time will allow the individual to develop a personal influence and to promote changes within the unit.

References and Recommended Reading

Department of Health, Nursing Division. (1989) *A Strategy for Nursing*. A Report of the Steering Committee, London.

Department of Health (1989) *Working for Patients* HMSO, London.

Nurses, Midwives and Health Visitors, Rules Approvals Orders. (1983) 873 HMSO, London.

Nurses, Midwives and Health Visitors (Midwives Training) Amendment Rules Approval Order. (1990) HMSO, London.

Report of an inquiry into the management of the health service to the Secretary of State. (1983) (The Griffiths Report). HMSO, London.

Chapter 4
Nursing research, computers in nursing, ward budgeting, presentation and analysis of data

The purpose of this chapter is to provide a basic introduction to the following subjects:

- Research in nursing
- Computers in nursing
- Ward budgets
- Presenting and analysing data.

Some nurses may feel that none of these topics is relevant for them and their practice, or at least that they have low priority. This chapter intends to provide some useful information for those nurses who are already interested in the subjects and might stimulate those who are not, to develop or participate in some new activities. Who knows, it might be fun!

Research in nursing

What do we mean by 'research in nursing'? In recent years some purists have tried to make distinctions between the various different types of research, indicating that nursing research is somehow intrinsically different from medical or scientific research. This may not be a helpful or necessary distinction. *The Shorter Oxford English Dictionary* defines research as 'investigation, inquiry into things' or 'the act of searching (closely or carefully) for or after a specified thing or person'. Does it matter who conducts the research or under what umbrella?

Research in nursing encompasses a variety of activities which may be undertaken by nurses or by others involved in the health care process. It includes 'nursing research' which is intended to mean research into the practice of nursing or into affairs which influence it. This kind of research may be carried out in clinical settings by clinical nurses or by academics. It may often be carried out by students of degree or higher degree programmes who have to carry out a piece of research for their qualification. These students should always be supervised to ensure that the research is valid (see Glossary) and appropriate to the setting. Small research studies may be undertaken by students taking other courses.

'Research in nursing' includes research conducted by other health professionals such as physiotherapists, speech therapists and doctors. This research is included here because nurses are often involved, particularly when patients are included in the study. Nurses may be needed to support patients, to ensure that they are adequately informed or to collect information or data. Nurses may be able to apply the research findings. Some medical researchers employ a nurse to take on these roles and also to coordinate data collection. These nurses are often in the lucky position of being able to undertake some research of their own while employed to assist in the research undertaken by others.

There are a number of other ways in which nurses become involved in research. These range from simple product evaluations to complex studies in quality assurance (see Chapter 5). Collecting information on a routine basis on things such as patient dependency levels or length of patient stay is a form of research in nursing and its value should not be underestimated.

Also included as an aspect of 'research in nursing' is the reading, appreciation, dissemination and application of research results. This may sound daunting, but the nurse who keeps up-to-date in her own field by critically reading appropriate journals and who shares the information she gleans, and tries to implement any new ideas, is involved in research and will stimulate a similar interest in others. It may be useful to introduce a regular ward meeting to discuss journal articles or books that have been read by members of the ward team, and to keep a file or files of relevant literature.

Why do we need research in nursing?

We must all have been impressed at some time in our professional lives by the wisdom and experience of ward sisters. If we could only catch the wisdom and write it down we would have a rich feast of concepts of nursing practice

McFarlane, 1977

Perhaps this is, in part, what research in nursing is attempting to do – to capture wisdom, write it down and develop generalizations from it so that it can be taught to the next generation of nurses.

In professional and academic terms though research is needed to:

- Provide a basis for decision-making at all levels of the profession
- Develop and refine nursing theories that serve as a guide to nursing practice and which can be organized into a body of scientific nursing knowledge
- Become an established profession.

Perhaps it would be useful to look at these responses in more detail and in less academic terms.

First, how do nurses make decisions in clinical practice? Most nurses would agree that a professional judgement may be made in one of three ways. These are:

(1) Tradition or intuition which does not necessarily involve thinking the problem through, but can be applied immediately
(2) Trial and error
(3) Using research findings based in a theoretical framework.

These ways can be used in combination and in different combinations in different situations. There are benefits and disadvantages associated with each of these ways of reaching a professional judgement and no one method is adequate on its own, but perhaps an examination of the pros and cons illustrated in Tables 4.1, 4.2 and 4.3 will help to back up the case for more nursing research.

Nursing has traditionally been taught by the bedside, but now much of a nurse's training time is spent in the classroom and clinical experience is likely to decrease with the advent of Project 2000. This means that much of the 'art' of nursing that used to be picked up on the job, must

Table 4.1   Methods of clinical decision-making: Trial and error

Pros	Cons
• Uses clinical experience	• Where do the ideas for 'trial' come from?
• Eventually produces a result that works	• It is haphazard, not logical in application
• Practice can change as new materials, equipment and knowledge become available	• May not be necessary to make the 'errors'
	• The solution reached is unique to the problem and may not work in all situations

Table 4.2   Methods of clinical decision-making: Tradition

Pros	Cons
• Survived the test of time • Practice is well established and accepted by nurses • Saves time and energy • Know it does no harm • Easy to pass on knowledge in clinical setting	• May be less willing to try new or alternative ways • Nurses may believe practice is the only way • Tend not to evaluate the outcome of practice • Cannot justify the use of the practice if asked or challenged • Practice does not change with the advent of new materials, equipment or knowledge

Table 4.3   Methods of clinical decision-making: Based on research findings

Pros	Cons
• Secure basis for decision making • Can be applied in any similar situation • Can justify decision • Make fewer 'errors' • Encourages critical thinking • Changes as new materials, equipment and knowledge become available	• Time-consuming • Not yet readily available • Not written in easily understandable way • Not yet enough research conducted into clinically applicable subjects

now be organized into a framework that can be discussed in the classroom and then applied in practice. Nursing research must therefore seek to develop theories which will provide this framework.

This is all very well, but still not a very meaningful or persuasive argument for sceptics. Table 4.4 provides some more concrete examples of why nursing research is needed to maximize the quality of patient care.

How do you 'do' research?

Learning how to do research need not be difficult and small studies may be undertaken with great ease, with validity (see Glossary) and speed. Most research, though, is complex because patients and nurses are people and don't necessarily obey neat rules. It is more difficult to study

Table 4.4   Practical reasons for needing nursing research

---

1   Patients receiving new treatments in medicine may require new nursing skills which need to be developed and tested.
2   As new equipment and materials become available, nursing knowledge must be updated, and nursing care changed to suit. Any changes should be evaluated logically.
3   Nurses aim to provide the maximum quality of patient care within the resources available. Research can help to ensure that care given is of high quality, because it increases nursing knowledge.
4   Research findings provide nurses with ammunition to fight for patient rights, e.g. the patient's need for preoperative information (Hayward 1975).
5   To solve specific problems.
6   The act of participating in research may maintain or improve nurse satisfaction and morale.

---

them as a result. This chapter does not intend to *teach* the reader how to do research and anyone wishing to pursue it is referred to the reading list at the end of the chapter. Whatever the scale of the research project, there must be a logical approach to solving the problem or to obtaining and analysing information. This is called the research process and it always follows the same stages as shown in Table 4.5.

For the nurse who wants to read research reports, some of the terminology may appear foreign, so a glossary of terms may be helpful and is included at the end of the chapter. The important thing to remember when reading research reports is that just because they contain the magic word 'research', this does not make them valid or significant. Nurses at any level must feel free to criticize research findings, and not accept them as read. Some of the things that often lead to criticism are shown in Table 4.6.

Table 4.5   The research process

---

1   Decide on a research problem
2   Review relevant literature
3   State aims and objectives of the research
4   Design the study and methods to be used
5   Construct instruments
6   Funding
7   Ethical considerations (submit to Ethical Committee)
8   Communication with all involved (written and verbal)
9   Pilot study
10   Data collection
11   Analysis
12   Presentation of findings

Table 4.6   Possible criticisms of research reports

---

1   Is the aim of the study clear?
2   What is the date of the study? Is it old work?
3   Does the method used seem appropriate for the research?
4   What is the sample size? Is it adequate?
5   How is the sample selected? Could this lead to bias?
6   Over how long and when was the study conducted? Is this an important issue in relation to the aims of the work?
7   Are the results presented clearly?
8   Would you draw the same conclusions as the writer from the results given?
9   Do the results contradict or confirm previous work?
10   Does further work need to be done to be sure the results are valid and reliable?
11   Can or should the results be applied in other settings?
12   What has this study added to nursing knowledge?

Some references for pieces of research that affect nursing practice are given in the recommended reading at the end of the chapter.

Computers in nursing

Many people think that computers are large, complex, totally incomprehensible and remote. Whether we like it or not, they are here to stay and the next decade or so may well see the biggest change ever to confront nurses and nursing – the use of computers in patient care.

At present within the NHS, computerization has begun to take over many of the clerical and administrative functions of the hospital. For example, the admissions department is usually computerized, with a database of patients waiting for admission. The outpatient appointment system is also usually computerized. Not only are computers used more and more in pathology, haematology and microbiology to analyse the samples for tests ordered by doctors, but the results are now also computerized, and may be easily viewed on a suitable computer terminal. These are but a few examples of how close computers are getting to nursing practice. Perhaps it is worth looking at how the future might bring them even closer to our personal professional practice. Indeed in some places, perhaps it already has.

Computers and nursing practice

Computer technology is currently in use in many units for the purposes of monitoring patients' cardiovascular and respiratory systems, usually in intensive or coronary care units. It is also used for monitoring the speed of delivery of intravenous fluids when this is a particularly important aspect of care. The nurse continues to assess, implement and evaluate, but more precise and accurate data are used due to computer technology.

The next step in development of computers in nursing must be the automation of the nursing process. If one looks to the United States of America for a foretaste of what's to come, the changes in the documentation of care and in communication seem to be the most dramatic. Perhaps presenting a scenario will be the best illustration of the changes that can be produced.

When a patient is admitted to a hospital ward, a staff nurse initiates the nursing assessment using a portable clipboard size computer terminal. When the assessment data are entered, the computer produces (on the screen) a selection of possible care plans appropriate to the assessment details. The nurse can then select the ones she needs and modifies the goals and interventions so that they are suitable for her patient. As the patient's condition changes, the nursing care plan can be revised and evaluated and a discharge plan can be devised and printed out for the patient to take home.

At the time for change of shift, the nursing care plan can be printed out including nursing actions to be taken if needed, and handed to the oncoming nurses. This ensures that omissions of communication are rare.

Medical staff enter all drug prescriptions directly into their patients' computerized records and the computer then alerts the nurse to observe for any side-effects or drug interactions. The computer also prints out a drug administration order at the appropriate time. In addition, the drug order is automatically printed out in the pharmacy department, so that if the drug is a non-stock item, the pharmacy can ensure that it is delivered to the ward before the time it is due. It is suggested that reductions in drug errors occur when a computerized system is implemented (Butler, 1978; Tamarisk, 1982).

Communication to all departments is enhanced by the ability of the computer to transmit orders to distant departments such as X-ray, haematology and pathology.

If the nurse is unsure about any aspect of patient care, she has access to computerized files regarding pharmacology, procedures, diseases and anything else selected to be included. Thus she can easily get up-to-date information to plan patient care.

Patient education material is also readily available and the computer can print out information to meet the needs of the patient and his family. It could not supplant the nurse, but could be a useful additional source of supportive information.

There are many questions that need to be raised and answered before attempting to implement such a system. These are mostly technical, legal, educational and ethical issues such as ensuring that access to computerized records is available only to the people who should have access to them, and who should those individuals be? Issues such as the legal problem of whether changing a nursing care plan, deleting the previous entry should be allowed. Should records be kept of every care plan printed out, or is it sufficient to save them in computer memory? The nurse who is to use the system must be educated in its use both prior to and during implementation. There is much work to be done before full computerization can take place.

This view of what can be possible using computers in clinical practice may still be a long way off in this country, but it almost certainly will come in time. It is important that nurses in Britain accept its inevitability and get involved in the planning of the systems we would like to use. It may not be advantageous to adopt the American model in its entirety but it could be useful to learn from it and adapt it to our needs.

Computers in nurse education

The role of computers in nurse education is already developing in this country. The computer plays a part initially in storing information about prospective candidates for a course of study, and in keeping records of existing students and their results. More and more complex curricula are being developed, and more and more students are enrolling for post-registration education. The computer is vital in developing and storing the information necessary to run all the courses now available. So the nurse teacher must consider developing her own computer literacy, and should be able to make use of the systems now available to aid curriculum planning and storage of information.

Within schools and colleges of nursing, computer programs are now available to assist in the teaching of some subjects. For example, programs are published by the Open Software Library (address in reference section) on topics such as drug calculations (Fish, E.J.), wound management (Morrison, D.) and off-duty rotas (Ward, S.) among many others.

At present, these packages are only used as an adjunct to teacher-led instruction, but as more become available student-led learning will become more common. This could involve the use of a computer in the student's home or workplace and employ distance learning techniques (Robinson, 1989). Through these methods, the student takes on a more responsible and accountable role for learning and is able to learn at her own pace in a non-threatening way. Silva (1973) paints a futuristic picture, but perhaps it is not too far from reality?

> The student will come to her computer terminal – located in her home – and select the learning package and the computer approach that is most congruous with her learning style, interests and goals at a given point in time. Accessible to her will be a wide variety of multimedia tools ... Computerised robots who can converse with her and who respond to a wide variety of symptoms and stresses ... will give her opportunities to experiment with ... nursing care prior to caring for people. (p. 94)

Computers in nursing administration

As hospitals generally become more computerized, so nursing administrators will need to develop their skills in dealing with computer technology. Many of the tasks that they are responsible for deal with information storage and retrieval which are supremely suited to computerization. Nurse managers could use the computer for the storage, analysis and interpretation of statistics related to patients or staff, such as bed occupancy, patient dependency, sickness rates or staff turnover.

Table 4.7 gives an indication of the functions that can be included in a computerized management system, but it must be remembered that these systems may not live up to expectations if they have been poorly designed, badly implemented or if the individuals using them lack confidence in their use.

Table 4.7 Functions that can be included in a computerized management system

1   Staff rostering
2   Absence, attendance and redeployment records
3   Agency and bank nurse working
4   Payment and pension details
5   Recruitment records
6   Wastage rates and reasons for leaving
7   Individual staff professional data
8   Individual staff personal data
9   Skill mix management
10 Manpower modelling and planning

Computers in nursing research

There is an obvious application for computers in research. Indeed, much research could not be carried out without the aid of computers to analyse the data. But the computer is also invaluable for data storage and to provide a database of, for example, patients involved in the study. The computer serves also as a word processor and as such enables easy production of research reports and other related material.

In summary, then, the computer is here to stay and will influence every aspect of the nursing world before long. In many areas, computer science is well developed, while in others, it still has a long way to go. Nurses must familiarize themselves with computer terminology and applications in order to participate in the development of appropriate software for their specific needs.

Ward budgeting

Initially, being asked to become the budgetholder for a unit may seem a very threatening and onerous task – perhaps the best avoided if possible. However, as it is likely to be a requirement of being in charge of the ward, some understanding of where the idea came from and how to go about developing a budget might be useful.

Where has it come from?

In her preface to the sixth report of the NHS/DHSS Health Services Information Steering Group, Mrs Korner wrote:

> The management of the NHS must at all times be able to demonstrate that the very large amount of public expenditure devoted to health care is properly spent, that funds are prudently allocated, expenditure strictly controlled, performance critically examined and competing claims for resources judiciously assessed.

The NHS has had cost and budgetary systems since its inception, but these have not been designed to keep track of the 'who, what, where and why' of expenditure. New cost accounting and budgeting systems have now been developed (Perrin, 1988) which, together with computerized information services, will enable the management of the NHS to:

(1) Distinguish precisely what has taken place and at what cost
(2) Forecast what is likely to happen and how much it is likely to cost

(3)   Introduce deliberate changes in the pattern of health care provision, knowing what the effects of such changes are likely to be

(4)   Provide staff with budgets based on defined levels of activity which they can positively control.

The introduction of budgeting in the clinical setting has been slow – partly due to resistance exhibited by the medical and paramedical professions and partly due to the limited finance available for the upgrading and computerization of activity and workload data which is essential for the running of a clinical budget. In addition, there are insufficient financial advisors or management accountants to cope with widespread development. Perrin (1988) states that it takes at least three or four years to introduce a working clinical management budget system in a hospital – little wonder then that it has been slow to become a widespread development.

Preparing a budget

There is no definitive plan for the implementation of management budgeting in the NHS. Each Health Authority is able to devise its own system (or variety of systems) based on Department of Health documents and its own needs.

The first steps in budgeting must be similar for everyone and a systematic approach will help. First, the backup and support systems must be in place:

- readily available information
- resource people
- authority to implement change
- evaluation and feedback
- formal and informal education.

Once these are established, the preparation of the budget can start. There are two basic approaches used to define the budget for an organization and its departments. These are incremental budgeting and zero-based budgeting.

Incremental budgeting has been the most common approach to budget setting in the NHS and involves taking the previous year's expenditure and adding to it or subtracting from it various allowances which may take into consideration:

(1)   Expected annual inflation

(2)   Planned changes in service levels

(3)   Planned service developments
(4)   Cost improvements achieved or expected
(5)   Previous overspending.

These allowances make up the 'increment' to the budget which may be different in each department, so reflecting clinical changes.

The major drawback of incremental budgeting is that it does not encourage managers to review existing standards of quality or productivity in planning the new budget.

Zero-based budgeting attempts to rectify this. As a starting point for the building of each budget it assumes zero activity, zero expenditure and zero income. Each element of activity or expenditure is then reviewed as to whether it is still valid and relevant. This is a time-consuming process if it is to be conducted properly. The learning programme 'Using Information in Managing the Nursing Resource' (Greenhalgh and Company, 1991) in the module on financial management suggests that there needs to be a balance between incremental budgeting and zero-based budgeting such that incremental budgeting is usually used but every 3–5 years zero-based budgeting is undertaken.

Whichever method of budgeting is used, Table 4.8 offers some suggestions for items that need to be considered in preparing the budget. Each service unit or department that has a budget defined for it is normally referred to as a 'cost centre' and each will usually have its own budget holder. Within each cost centre, items of expenditure are referred to in groups or 'expense categories' which may be referred to as 'expense codes'. Ideally, the expense codes used will be the same across the institution but each unit may need to have access to one or more unique codes for items of expenditure which are unique to that unit. Examples of expense categories are shown in Table 4.9.

Table 4.8   Items to be considered in preparing a budget

---

1   What staff are needed to provide agreed levels/quality of care?
2   Are there any changes in skill mix or care requirements expected in the year ahead?
3   What improvements or savings could be made in current working practices?
4   What information is available for the current year?
5   Are there any errors in this information (such as incorrect staff costs allocated to the ward or incorrect stock issues)?
6   Are there variations during the year in levels of activity or expenditure?
7   Should the consequent variation in expenditure be averaged out over the year?
8   How detailed should the budget be?
9   At what level of detail will expenditure be monitored against the budget?
10 Do plans need to be made for unforseen costs (for example, the costs of recruiting and training new staff if current staff leave)?

Table 4.9	Examples of expense categories

1	Staff costs including overtime and special duty payments
2	Salary related costs (e.g. superannuation)
3	Drugs
4	Dressings
5	Linen
6	Laundry
7	Uniforms
8	CSSD
9	Maintenance and servicing of equipment
10	Stationery
11	Telephone
12	Crockery and cutlery
13	Catering and food supplies

There are other ways of breaking down the information included in a budget which may make it more useful at managerial level. These involve looking at the various costs and describing them in different ways. Examples of these include direct and indirect costs, fixed and variable costs, overheads. Definitions of these terms can be found in the glossary at the end of the chapter.

Once a draft budget has been established it is submitted to the accountants who will develop a master budget for the whole organization. This is then reviewed against the total anticipated income and individual budget-holders will then be asked to adjust their draft budgets accordingly.

The consequences for the sister or charge nurse

Although becoming a budget holder may seem to be yet another time-consuming, clerical activity, it is hoped that the information provided above gives a good idea of some of the bonuses for the sister or charge nurse. Instead of having change imposed by managers, the nurse budget-holder is in a position to influence the direction of change and to monitor the effect it has. The management of the unit really does lie in the hands of the budget-holder rather than with a more distant manager.

One of the reasons for developing unit budgets is to ensure value for money and to produce cost improvements. When planning the introduction of ward budgeting, the organization should decide how to provide incentives or rewards for cost saving. The sister or charge nurse then has the pleasure of distributing these rewards.

Of course not all the consequences will be positive ones. There is no doubt that, at least initially, preparing a budget is time-consuming and involves mountains of computer printout and interpreting tables. It may also involve scrutinizing current practices. Wanda Shafer (1991) reports:

> Once I knew what was on the shelves and in what quantities, it was possible to question the effect if stocks were reduced; asking such questions as:
> - How long does it take to process an order?
> - What procedure would the ward follow if they ran out of an item?

Once the budget is prepared and accepted, the work does not stop there. Every month a budget statement arrives on the budget-holder's desk to enable him/her to determine if the budget is being adhered to, and if not, why not. At the end of the year, the analysis of the year's budget must be thorough to enable the development of a new one.

Presenting and analysing data

One of the main functions of managers is to take decisions. To perform this function effectively they require information. The definition of 'statistics' as given by *The Shorter Oxford English Dictionary* is: 'numerical facts or data collected and classified'. So the collection and use of statistics must be a part of every ward manager's job, providing the information needed to take fully informed decisions. Examples of some statistics that are commonly collected are:

- Types of patients admitted to the ward
- Staffing levels on the ward
- Rate of hospital-acquired infection
- Level of bed occupancy.

Of course, the advent of the computer has meant that the collection of these statistics is much simpler and less time-consuming but it is still important that all data collected are valid, appropriate, accurate, up-to-date and timely (meaning that the information is supplied in time for action to be taken). Crucial to all of these is that the data are understandable and presented and analysed in such a way that they can be clearly and easily understood. Without 'understanding' how can the validity and appropriateness of the data be assessed and how can informed decisions be taken?

This section of the chapter aims to provide some help in understanding the numerical data that ward managers might be faced with and a glossary of terms is included at the end of the chapter. A detailed description of statistics and the analysis of data cannot be given in a book of this size, but the interested reader can find more information from books in the Recommended Reading list.

Data can be presented in a variety of ways – tables, graphs, bar charts and diagrams. The aim of presenting data in these ways is to summarize and clarify the information, to make it more easily understandable. When reading or writing reports, it is useful to know the main features of tables and charts and the advantages and disadvantages of each.

Tables

The first thing that needs to be done with newly collected data is to put them into some kind of format that can be more easily reviewed. The easiest way is to put them into a table. There are a variety of ways in which this can be done, examples of which are shown in Tables 4.10 and 4.11.

Table 4.10 shows the basic features of all tables. To ensure clarity it has:

- A title
- Headings for columns (and rows if appropriate)
- The source of the data indicated, which lends credibility to the figures (not shown in these examples)
- A table number so that reference can easily be made to it in the text
- Readable data items.

Table 4.11 has all the basic features described above, but in addition, some analysis of the figures is done to enable easy interpretation of the

Table 4.10 The length of stay of 27 patients following varicose vein surgery

Length of stay	Number of patients
1 Day	8
2 Days	11
3 Days	3
4 Days	0
5 Days	3
6 Days	0
7 Days	0
8 Days	1
9 Days	0
10 Days	0
11 Days	0
12 or more Days	1

Table 4.11   Hospital admissions in one year by speciality and patient type

Speciality	Inpatients	Day cases	All cases
General surgery	6 000	4 000	10 000
General medicine	6 000	2 000	8 000
Orthopaedics	2 000	1 000	3 000
Obstetrics	1 000	0	1 000
Gynaecology	2 500	500	3 000
Geriatrics	5 000	0	5 000
Total	**22 500**	**7 500**	**30 000**

raw data. The total number of inpatient and day cases in each speciality is worked out, so that comparisons between the specialities can be made. Also, the total number of inpatients and the total number of day cases has been computed together with the total number of cases in all specialities. With these figures, it is easy to see, for example, that the majority of patients were admitted for general surgery (10 000 of 30 000) but that nearly half of these were day cases. Further, more detailed analysis can be carried out on these data, such as working out the percentage of inpatients in each speciality. The analysis required depends on the reason for collecting the data in the first place.

There are a large number of statistical tests that can be carried out on data, but this chapter cannot hope to cover them. Some are mentioned in the glossary and further information can be found in the texts given in the Recommended Reading list at the end.

Graphs, charts and diagrams

Graphs, charts and diagrams are usually used to represent information in a way that aids interpretation. Although exact figures may be shown, it is usually more difficult to determine the exact data figures. These ways of presenting information are usually used for clarity when summarizing data or for illuminating comparisons.

Table 4.12 shows some budget details in table form. Figure 4.1 shows the same data arranged in a bar chart. Although it is more difficult to determine the exact expenditure for each item, it is much easier to compare relative costs when looking at the bar chart.

Figure 4.1 also shows some of the important features of all charts and diagrams:

Table 4.12 Sample expenditure for one year for a general surgical unit

Item of expenditure	Actual expenditure (£s)
Provisions	958
Dressings	1 112
Other medicines and supplies	604
Surgical gloves	300
Drainage bags and sets	350
Other consumables	526
Medical equipment <£1000	364
Appliances	500
General catering	480
Disposables	200
Incontinence materials	220
Paper towels	285

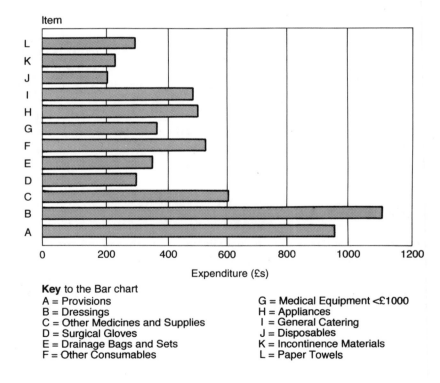

Key to the Bar chart
A = Provisions
B = Dressings
C = Other Medicines and Supplies
D = Surgical Gloves
E = Drainage Bags and Sets
F = Other Consumables
G = Medical Equipment <£1000
H = Appliances
I = General Catering
J = Disposables
K = Incontinence Materials
L = Paper Towels

Fig. 4.1 Sample expenditure for one year for a general surgical unit, (bar chart presentation)

- A title
- Axes labels explaining what is being measured or represented by each axis. The horizontal axis is known as the x-axis and the vertical is the y-axis.
- Axis markers which mark out the values used in the diagram
- Shadings to clearly represent different categories
- Keys or legends to explain the different shadings or labels used in the diagram.

There are many ways of arranging data in diagrammatic form, ranging from a simple bar-chart like that shown, to more complex multiple bar-charts and multiple line graphs. The choice of which way to present data is determined by which variables are of interest and in what detail the data must be retrievable from the diagram. Whether preparing a report or reading it, it is of value to remember that tables and graphs are intended to provide illustrations of the text, and, in some cases, proof of a stated conclusion. If the table or graph is so complex that it cannot be easily interpreted then it has little use.

Summary

This chapter has tried to provide a brief introduction to some of the new challenges facing ward sisters and charge nurses in the 1990s. It would be impossible to provide detailed information on all the subjects covered, so an attempt has been made to enable the reader to reach a broad understanding of the topic and its terminology, and to provide a source of further information for those especially interested.

Glossary

Abstract   usually at the beginning of a research report or article, this provides a summary of why the study was done and the main results.

Bias   a distortion of the findings as a result of an unwanted influence (see Observer bias).

Classification   the placing of data with similar features into specified unambiguous categories.

Chi–Square Test   a test to determine whether a difference in the results from what would have been expected could be due to chance, or whether it is a 'significant' (i.e. 'real') difference.

Control group   a group of research subjects who do not experience the factor under consideration so that a comparison can be made with the results obtained in the experimental group.

Cohort   a group of subjects who are studied over a period of time.

Data   pieces of recorded information, facts or phenomena resulting from research.

Database   a filing system for organizing, sorting, retrieving, transcribing and processing data.

Demographic data   information about the personal characteristics of all the individuals under study.

Dependent variable   the aspect being studied to determine whether the experimental factor (the independent variable) has an effect.

Direct costs   are those that can be controlled directly by the budget-holder and/or staff working for him or her.

Experimental group   a group of research subjects who *do* experience the factor under consideration so that a comparison can be made with the results obtained in the control group.

Fixed costs   those components of the total cost of a service which do not alter over a period of time.

Hardware   the physical components of the computer: the screen, keyboard, printer, and internal components or link-up to a central computer.

Hypothesis   a statement of a relationship based on knowledge, information or observation but which has not yet been proved or disproved.

Independent variable   the experimental factor which is deliberately manipulated to assess its effect (e.g. given to the experimental group and not the control group).

Indirect costs   usually these represent the cost charged to a department for services supplied by another (e.g. X-rays). The unit cost (for each X-ray) is not in the direct control of the budget-holder.

Interview
  structured: an interview which is conducted using set questions and a determined range of possible responses;
  semi-structured: an interview which is conducted to answer set questions but allows some flexibility both in the questioning and in the range of responses;
  unstructured: an interview about a specific topic but which allows spontaneous questions and free responses.

Literature review   a brief summary of related published work.

Mean   the average value.

Median   the number which occurs in the middle of a sequence of scores.

Mode   the score that occurs most frequently in a range of scores.

Methodology   how data is to be/was collected and analysed in order to answer the research question. The methodology must be specified and must include information relating to the sample size and how it is to be selected, and details of any research tools to be used.

Non-participant observation   research method in which situations are observed when the observer is not involved.

Null hypothesis   a negative hypothesis – a statement that there will be no observable relationship in the results (i.e. the experiment will not work).

Observer bias   bias that occurs when two observers, viewing the same situation, unintentionally but systematically record different results.

Overhead costs   costs borne by the organization which cannot sensibly be apportioned to individual budgets (e.g. maintenance of grounds).

Participant observation   a research method in which situations are observed while the observer is taking part.

Pilot study   a preliminary study carried out to test the methods and tools intended to be used in the main study.

Population   the complete group of people or things (individuals, hospitals, medical records etc.) which could be selected as subjects of a research project.

Probability (p)   the likelihood of an event happening by chance, rather than being a direct result of the experiment. p is expressed numerically on a scale from 0 to 1. A finding which is indicated as having a probability of less than 0.01 ($p < 0.01$) means that it was likely to have occurred by chance in fewer than 1 in 100 instances.

Random sampling   systematic selection of a sample to ensure that all members of a population stand an equal chance of being selected.

Reliability   whether or not the same test will give the same results when used under the same conditions on different occasions or by different researchers.

Research tool   any instrument used in the collection of data. Tools may be in the form of a questionnaire, interview schedule, observation record chart or a combination of these.

Response rate   proportion of those approached to participate in a study who fully completed the exercise.

Sample   a selection of people or things from the total population, to be subjects for a research project.

Software   any program, together with any procedures, rules or instruction manuals necessary to run the program.

Standard deviation   a measure of the spread of a distribution of results – an indication of how much each result varies from the mean of all the results.

Statistical significance   whether or not statistical tests can show that an observed difference between experimental results and those from the control group (or those predicted by the original hypothesis) is 'real' (i.e. unlikely to be a chance finding).

Validity   whether or not a test measures what it is supposed to measure.

Variable   any factor, characteristic or attribute of a population which varies from one individual to the next and so may be used to distinguish one from another for the purposes of study (examples are patients' age, sex, diagnosis etc).

Variable costs   those elements of a total cost which are more responsive to a change in demand.

References

Butler, E.A. (1978) An automated hospital information system *Nursing Times*, **74**, 245–7.

Greenhalgh & Company (1991) (in conjunction with a five regional consortium) *Using Information in Managing the Nursing Resource* Crown Copyright, Greenhalgh & Co Ltd.

Hayward, J.C. (1975) *Information – a prescription against pain* Royal College of Nursing, London.

Korner, E. (1984) (see NHS/DHSS, 1984).

Little, W., Fowler, H.W. and Coulson, J. (1983) *The Shorter Oxford English Dictionary* 3rd Edition, OUP, London.

McFarlane, J.K. (1977) Developing a theory of nursing *Journal of Advanced Nursing*, **2(3)**, 261–70.

NHS/DHSS (1984) Steering Group on Health Services Information *Sixth Report* (on the collection and use of financial information). HMSO.

Open Software Library, 164 Windsor Road, Ashton-in-Makerfield, Wigan, WN4 9ES. Tel: 0942-712385.

Perrin, J. (1988) *Resource Management in the NHS*, Chapman and Hall, London.

Robinson, K. (1989) *Open and Distance Learning for nurses*, Longman UK.

Shafer, W. (1991) Managing a budget at ward level. *Professional Nurse* August 1991.

Silva, M.C. (1973) Nursing education in the computer age. *Nursing Outlook*, **21**, 94–8.

Tamarisk, N.K. (1982) The computer as a clinical tool. *Nursing Management*, **13**, 46–9.

Recommended Reading

Cormack, D.F.C. (1984) *The research process in nursing* Blackwell Scientific Publications, Oxford.

Clark, J.M. and Hockey, L. (1979) *Research for Nursing – A guide for the enquiring nurse*, HM&M publishers.

Distance Learning Centre (1988) *Research Awareness (series of 13 modules)*, DLC, South Bank Polytechnic, Crown Copyright.

Greenhalgh & Company (1991) (in conjunction with a five regional consortium) *Using Information in Managing the Nursing Resource* Crown Copyright, Greenhalgh & Co Ltd.

Hockey, L. (1985) *Nursing Research - Mistakes and Misconceptions*, Churchill-Livingstone, Edinburgh.

Ogier, M.E. (1982) *An Ideal Sister?*, Royal College of Nursing, London.

Ogier, M.E. (1989) *Reading Research*, Scutari Press, London.

Orton, H.D. (1981) *Ward Learning Climate*, Royal College of Nursing, London.

Perrin, J. (1988) *Resource Management in the NHS*, Chapman and Hall, London.

Reid, N.G. and Boore, J.R. (1987) *Research Methods and Statistics in Health Care*, Edward Arnold, London.

Wilson Barnett, J.C. (ed.) (1983) *Nursing Research – Ten studies in Patient Care*, John Wiley and Sons, Chichester.

Chapter 5
Quality in nursing

'Nursing audit', 'Quality assurance', 'Quality of care', 'Setting standards', these phrases are now frequently in the nursing press and on nurses' and nurse managers' lips. They often conjure up images of an unwanted evil – 'Big Brother is watching us'; 'they're not going to be happy with what they find'; 'they're going to make us change the way we work', or similar. This chapter intends to provide nurses with information about what quality assurance is, why we need it, how to go about doing it and how best to use the results for the benefit of the nurses and patients on the ward. It also aims to dispel some of the fears and anxieties associated with quality assurance at ward level.

Definitions

There are a vast number of terms used in the literature about quality in nursing. This has led to some confusion about the meaning and implication of each. This section will attempt to clarify these terms.

The *Shorter Oxford English Dictionary* (1983) defines 'audit' as:

> an official examination of accounts (or activities) with verification by reference to witnesses and vouchers.

Recently, the NHS Management Executive (1991) have produced a Framework of Audit for Nursing Services (Project 32). In this document, Nursing Audit is defined as:

> Part of the cycle of quality assurance. It incorporates the systematic and critical analyses by nurses, midwives and health visitors, in conjunction with other staff, of the planning, delivery and evaluation of nursing and midwifery care, in terms of their use of resources and the outcomes for patients/clients, and introduces change in response to that analysis.

How is this different from quality assurance? 'Quality assurance in nursing' is about assuring clients of the quality of the nursing care they receive. It is about setting standards of quality for practice and monitoring how well those standards are met. It is directly related to patient care.

In contrast, audit is about monitoring all aspects of the supply and delivery of care, not just the quality. Project 32 suggests that there are six audit areas:

(1) Clinical care
(2) Workload management
(3) Deployment
(4) Personnel management
(5) Organizational arrangements
(6) Environment and support.

Within these areas there will be a range of categories and issues to be addressed. Audit is not exclusive to nursing, but can be applied as medical audit, pathology audit or any other group.

One aspect of quality assurance is the measurement of the quality of nursing care given to patients. In audit terms this could be called 'nursing care audit' (as opposed to 'nursing audit' which incorporates auditing all aspects of nursing).

The measurement of quality can only be done if nurses have some kind of working understanding of what 'quality' is.

Quality is a concept that is difficult to define. The *Chambers Dictionary* (1980) says:

quality is that which makes a thing what it is; nature, character, attitude; grade of goodness; excellence.

This does not help much if a nurse is trying to measure quality.

The World Health Organization (WHO, 1986) states:

Quality is ... the comparison of how the level of care actually provided compares with that which is defined as the wanted level of care.

The wanted level of care may be defined by anyone, but is frequently a political decision. The World Health Organisation (*op. cit*) suggests that quality is often calculated at the level above which care would be costly and below which it would be dangerous. This is reflected in the Griffiths Report (1983; see Chapter 3) which advocates a cost-effective health service, with value for money for the consumer and the provision of the best possible standards of care.

The quality of nursing care cannot itself be directly measured because it is not an absolute concept and different people may have different perspectives and expectations which make up their idea of 'quality'. In order to assess quality, it is broken down into component parts which reflect elements of the quality of care provided. These component parts are called 'standards'.

Standard is defined by the *Chambers Dictionary* (1980) as:

> a basis for measurement, an established or accepted model; a definite level of excellence or adequacy required, aimed at or possible.

The Royal College of Nursing states:

> A standard is the professionally agreed level of performance appropriate to the population addressed, which is observable, achievable, measurable and desirable.
>
> (RCN, 1986)

Any instrument (or tool) which is used to measure the quality of nursing care may take a variety of different forms but all will produce a figure or score of quality. An instrument maybe in the form of a questionnaire or survey or just a simple check-list. Every instrument should include instructions as to how and where it should be used, how to work out the score and how to interpret the results. Some existing instruments will be described later.

Why do nurses need quality assurance?

Concern about the quality of health care has been around for a long time. Florence Nightingale's *Notes on Nursing* (1858) is one of the best known examples relating specifically to nursing and a caring environment. More recently, WHO (European region) has published *Targets for Health for All* (1984), one of which states that:

> by 1990, all member states should have built effective mechanisms for ensuring quality of patient care within their health care systems.

The Griffiths Report has had considerable impact on the health service in this regard. The advent of a business-style management structure which may not include any nurses at the higher levels means that nurses must learn to present their needs and anxieties in a more tangible way. The results of measuring quality may provide a way to do this. If nurses fail to monitor their own performance, management may try to do it for them, at unit or regional level, or nationally.

The United Kingdom Central Council for Nursing, Midwifery and Health Visiting (UKCC, 1984) has laid down a code of conduct for the professional nurse which emphasizes the need for individual account-ability for decisions and actions. The Royal College of Nursing has set up a Standards of Care project which aims to carry out research to establish the theories and framework for measuring the quality of care, and also to provide practical guidelines for nurses at every level to enable them to maintain standards of care.

More recently, the National Health Service and Community Care Act (1990) has allowed the development of an internal market and the introduction of contracts for healthcare services. Together with this it has extended the remit of the Audit Commission to cover Health Authorities. The Act now requires all units to define precisely what purchasers can expect for their money and encourages purchasers to place contracts with those units which can demonstrate high quality, cost-effective treatment and care.

In summary then, nurses are under a great deal of pressure from a variety of political and professional sources to assure the quality of nursing care. There are two other important factors that may help to persuade any nurses who remain unconvinced. First, they have a responsibility to their patients to ensure that they are provided with the highest level of care, within nurses' control. Quality is not an absolute concept, different people may have different perspectives and expectations of quality. So each individual nurse may believe that she has high standards, but without some method of measuring quality, she cannot assure her patients of her own standards nor be sure that her colleagues have equally high standards.

Second, a common cry from the NHS workforce in this time of financial stringencies is: 'We can't take any more cutbacks – we are stretched to the limit.'. Perhaps nurses should be learning the skills to assess the effects of financial cutbacks on the quality of the care the patients receive to arm themselves with evidence of any deterioration resulting from such changes. They may then be in a position to argue for increases, or at least no further decreases, in resources and manpower.

How to set up a quality assurance programme

Few ward sisters or charge nurses will feel capable of setting up a quality assurance programme on their own. The information in this section is

provided to indicate where nurses who are interested in quality measurement might go to find others who are already involved. It also
provides a starting point and some guidance for nurses who are starting
up a programme at ward or unit level, or even throughout the hospital.

In many health districts there will be a committee responsible for all
quality assurance activities at district level. Below this level, there is no
uniform activity. Indeed there is great variation in what individual
hospitals and units are doing towards the same aim. However, if the
programme is to be effective, there are certain steps that should not be
ignored.

First, there should be a steering committee, the role of which is to
develop the programme together with the methods to be used and to
support the staff and others likely to be influenced by the work itself or
its results. The membership of the steering committee will vary from
place to place, but if the programme is to work with minimal antagonism
from staff, then a bottom-upwards approach to communication should
be adopted, supported throughout the hierarchy and this should be
reflected in the membership. Running a quality assurance programme
can be a costly business. One of the first things the committee will have
to do is to look at how much finance they can obtain and where from.
This may, in part, dictate the methods to be used.

The next step for the members of the steering committee must be to
identify the institutional philosophy and then develop their own values
and philosophy for nursing. Conflicts can easily arise when the institutional philosophy differs from that of the individual unit, so these need to
be ironed out at an early stage.

For example, nurses on a coronary care unit might identify a need for
the development of patient relaxation techniques such as massage or
aromatherapy. The nurses on this unit might develop a standard for care
which includes the use of patient relaxation techniques. If the institution
does not see this kind of work as a valuable use of nursing time, they will
oppose the training of nurses in these areas and may not provide the
finance to support it in terms of education, manpower or equipment. The
nurses would then fail to meet this particular standard, and be unable to
change their behaviour in order to do so. This kind of difference in
philosophical viewpoint needs to be addressed before the real work of
quality assurance begins.

Once the philosophy has been developed, the objectives for the
programme can be identified and a plan of action developed. The plan
must include descriptions of the methods to be used, who by and how
often. It must include information regarding communication channels to
all involved, accountability for planned actions and confidentiality of
results. There must be a proposed timetable not only for the implemen-

tation of the programme, but also for the feedback of results and for the implementation of resultant changes. A proposal for the education of staff involved as well as for their support needs to be included.

Methods of assuring quality

There are as many different methods of assuring quality as there are quality assurance groups. Examples that are widely used include:

- Peer review
- Questionnaires (patient and staff)
- Sample surveys
- Direct observation of staff and/or patients
- Self-recording by staff of what is done
- Statistical evaluation against predefined standards
- Spot checks (on data or records)
- Trend analyses
- Comparative analyses.

(NHS Management Executive, 1991)

Generally, there are three options from which to choose. Probably the easiest way is to use an already established quality monitoring tool. Some of those available will be discussed in greater detail later, but all have the disadvantage that the standards of care are prescribed by the people who developed the tool and these may not be appropriate to all settings or for the method of delivery of nursing care used on a specific unit. In addition, it may be expensive to buy the instrument and its accompanying workbook.

The second option is to modify an already established instrument to suit the needs of a particular unit. This has the disadvantage that the reliability of the tool may be reduced by the changes made to it, and so reliability tests need to be included in a pilot study.

The third option is to start from scratch and design an instrument or method specific to a particular department, unit or hospital. Many nurses new to quality assurance may not feel that they can attempt this without more expert help, and it also has the drawback of being very time-consuming.

In order to decide which is the best option, it may be a good idea to start by doing some reading of other people's experiences. Most nursing libraries now have the facility to do a literature search and will help in finding any literature needed. Some of the questions that the steering group need to consider include the following:

(1) Cost: it is cheap (in terms of ready cash, but not necessarily in time) to produce your own tool and may be expensive to use an existing one.
(2) Preparation time may be a consideration. If results are wanted quickly it may be better to use an existing tool.
(3) Is there a tool which is appropriate to the setting?
(4) Are patient dependency studies* included in the instrument and if not, are they needed?
(5) Is the scoring system appropriate? If scored manually, are the people with appropriate skills available? If scoring is to be done by computer, is it, and the people to use it, available?
(6) Who is to monitor quality? This is a great debate! Employing an outside evaluator ensures greater objectivity but may be costly and may be considered a greater threat by nursing staff. Using local staff ensures that the results are accepted as valid by the unit and acceptance of ensuing change may be easier but the objectivity of the observers may be questioned.
(7) Some instruments require a large number of observers to be available at one time. Is this possible? Is it possible to have the observers available at the times of day required by the instrument?

*Patient dependency studies involve the daily collection of information relating to the level of dependence on nursing care for every patient in the unit. The level of dependence is worked out using a formula based on the number and type of nursing activities required. The levels are usually from 1 to 4 or 5, with 1=low dependence or self caring and 4 or 5 = totally dependent or unconscious. Using this information, it can be seen when wards are busy or quiet and daily, weekly, monthly or annual trends can be observed.

Using an existing tool for measuring quality of nursing care

Some of the commonly used quality measurement tools are described and some of the advantages and disadvantages of each system are noted. This is not intended to provide sufficient information on which to make the decision as to which tool to choose, but merely to exemplify the range available and to act as an introductory guide to those unfamiliar with quality measurement.

The Rush Medicus Quality Monitoring Methodology for Nursing Care

The Rush Medicus Methodology (Hegyvary and Haussmann, 1975) is probably the best known and most widely used methodology in the world. It was developed in America in 1972 and has been extensively tested to demonstrate its reliability and validity (for a definition of these terms see Glossary at the end of Chapter 4) in that country. It uses a classification of patients by their level of self-sufficiency and each quality criterion in the methodology is coded as to the type of patient to which it can be applied. There are a total of 357 criteria divided into 32 sub-objectives and 6 main objectives. The criteria are available for a variety of clinical settings. From the master list of criteria, observation worksheets are produced by computer with 30–50 observations each. The sources of information are from direct observation of the patient, his environment, the nurses, their environment and management, as well as from patient and nurse interviews.

Quality is to be monitored 3 times a year on 10 per cent of patients and observations are to be taken at all times of the day and night.

Monitor – an Index of the Quality of Nursing Care for Acute Medical and Surgical Wards

Monitor (Goldstone *et al.*, 1984) is an adaptation for the United Kingdom of the Rush Medicus methodology described above. The tool is easy to use and comes with a detailed manual in which recommendations are made for how to go about the whole quality assurance exercise. The authors suggest that the instrument should be used once a year and that two observers carry out the evaluation procedure.

Monitor uses a patient dependency classification system and four separate questionnaires are available, each relating to a different patient dependency. In addition, there is a ward-based questionnaire which looks at the caring environment and at safety. The scoring system is easy and can be done manually. There are Monitor tools now available for a variety of different settings, including the community.

Monitor has been used extensively in Britain and has found a mixed response from its users. Some of the concerns are:

(1) Large number of questions for very ill patients (22 for a maximum dependency patient) (Kemp and Richardson, 1990).
(2) Document is tiring and time-consuming to use (Kemp and Richardson).
(3) May not be suitable for units that employ a task allocation method of delivery of care (Barnett and Wainwright, 1987).
(4) There may be a large number of non-applicable responses which reduces the number of applicable questions and hence may reduce the validity of the results in a specific section (Brittle and Marsh, 1986).

(5) Inter-observer reliability may be questioned particularly if obser-
     vers are not adequately prepared or familiar with the document
     (Brittle and Marsh, 1986; Whelan, 1987).

However, Monitor does provide an easy and accessible method of
measuring the quality of care.

Criteria for Care

The developers of Monitor have also developed a system for nurse
manpower planning called 'Criteria for Care' (Ball, Goldstone and
Collier, 1984). This system is intended to be used in conjunction with
Monitor and aims to provide a means of assessing the workload on
medical and surgical wards and the demand that such a workload places
on the nursing staff. It also provides a means of assessing the level of
care provided by nurses at any time of the day or night and on all days of
the week. The tool requires that patient dependency levels are studied
for at least six months in order to ascertain the average workload on a
particular unit.

Criteria for Care enables managers to make decisions about staffing
levels in full knowledge of how changes may affect the workload on a
given unit. It is an expensive tool to use in terms of the numbers of
observers required for a whole week of evaluation and for 24 hours a day
but it provides a vast amount of information about what nurses do and
when they do it, together with information about what care patients
receive and when they get it. The tool is complex to use but it is not
difficult to analyse the results.

Qualpac – the quality patient care scale

Qualpac (Wandelt and Ager, 1974) is an American tool but has now been
widely used in many settings in Britain. Nevertheless, each group that
uses it must ensure that the standards it prescribes reflect the culture
and quality expected of nurses in their own environment. It does not use
a patient dependency rating but patients are randomly selected and a
total of 15 per cent (minimum five patients) are observed. The instrument provides 68 items divided into six sections of nursing care type
(such as physical or communication). Each item is explained using cues
and a score is given on a five-point scale ranging from poorest to best
care. Observers spend two hours in direct observation of the care being
given and about one hour examining records.

Kemp and Richardson (1990) comment that this tool calls on observers to make value judgements which can be difficult when there are

many activities occurring at the same time and can easily lead to observer bias. They also state that in their opinion, 'it is the best scale available for observing how nurses react to the needs of patients particularly in the area of communication' (p. 67).

The PA Nursing Quality Measurement Scale

The PA Scale (PA, 1987) was developed by a management consultancy organization using nursing and health care consultants to design it. The management consultancy provide the in-service training, preparation of staff and the training of observers. The tool is divided into five sections which evaluate the workload and facilities available, the physical and human resources, the care given, the patients' views and finally makes recommendations for change in either care or resources. This tool is relatively new and as yet has received little attention in nursing literature. It appears to be relatively easy to use and leaves little room for value judgements.

If the steering group decides to use an existing tool, it has to be piloted to ensure that it suits the unit and that it is valid and reliable in the setting. Piloting the tool means trying it out on a small scale, not intending to measure quality, but to test the tool and the arrangements for using it. Observers should be prepared prior to the pilot study and tests carried out to ensure that all observers score in the same way (inter-observer reliability). Following the pilot study, the steering group must feel free to change their minds entirely or to make modifications as necessary.

Modifying an existing tool

This is considered by some to be the best option for measuring quality of care as it ensures that the tool is suitable for use within the specific institution without the problems inherent in producing a unique instrument. However, it is fraught with complications. It is not difficult to remove some questions from a questionnaire, but it is important to then address the effect that this has on the scoring and analysis of results – particularly when different questions or sections carry a different weight in terms of their score. Adding additional questions is similarly difficult, and also leads to problems of validity: does the new question measure quality in the same way as the others, or does it measure something slightly different? New questions also have to be tested for reliability, to ensure that they are not ambiguous and that observers will respond to them in the same way in a given situation. This is particularly true when value judgements are required and these questions are best avoided as much as possible.

Altering the wording of existing questions is usually permitted to some extent, if it ensures that the observers have a better understanding of the question, but altering wording can alter the meaning of the question so careful testing needs to be carried out.

As before, pilot work must be carried out thoroughly to ensure that the new tool works as intended, and that the scores are valid. Piloting an altered tool needs to be done much more thoroughly than when using an existing tool that has not been altered.

Developing a tool or method of measuring quality of care

There are advantages and disadvantages to developing a tool or methodology at local level. The benefits are that it will reflect local needs and culture and it will be owned by the group who will feel a sense of achievement in the work. This also means that the results of the work will be accepted by the group and by the rest of the staff more readily than if it were done using an existing tool or by outsiders.

The disadvantages are that it is very time-consuming to get it right and considerable piloting of any tool is required to ensure validity and reliability. It also means that each group to a greater or lesser extent, 're-invents the wheel' – time and effort that could perhaps be better spent. Others would argue that purely attempting to look at the issue of quality assurance and to develop a measurement tool, in itself can raise standards and morale (Dunn, 1990).

There are innumerable ways of monitoring the quality of nursing care without using a pre-existing tool. Some of these will be briefly described followed by a more detailed description of methods of setting standards and monitoring outcomes.

Phaneuf's Nursing Audit

Phaneuf's audit was developed in America. Phaneuf (1976) developed a scale of 50 items relating to nursing functions. Every month, a committee made up of nurses from all levels and settings, reviews a specified number of nursing records, chosen randomly from the notes of patients discharged the previous month. A score is given for each of the 50 items. After the audit, a report is submitted to the administrator, with recommendations, and the administrator must respond in writing to the committee. This method of monitoring quality is easily developed for use in any unit or department and provides minimal threat to staff. It does, however, have the disadvantage of using only nursing records, which do not necessarily reflect the quality of nursing care, but may only monitor nurses' abilities to write notes! It also means that if nurses know that this is being done (as they should!), they may spend more time on writing up their notes, and consequently, less time on patient care.

Quality Circles

A small group of staff, which may be representative of all disciplines and from the same work area, meet regularly to present, discuss and solve problems related to their work. These problems may be related directly to a particular patient, but need not be. The group should be led by a properly trained facilitator and may be more productive if management is represented.

This method is more of a quality monitoring system than a measurement of quality, and as such it is difficult to make comparisons over time. One cannot say that quality has improved or decreased except in an intuitive way, unless there are figures to back it up.

Performance appraisal systems

These are now used throughout the Health Service. Whatever system of appraisal is used, be it peer review or structured interview or anything else, it should serve as a method of monitoring quality. No comparisons can be made resulting from the lapse of time nor from introduced change, except in an intuitive way, as no scores are given. Also, these methods relate only to individual nurses, not the function of the group as a whole – meaning that the quality of care given on the unit cannot be inferred from the results of individual appraisal.

The development of measurable standards of care

This has become a common way of addressing the issue of quality at unit level. Close (1990) describes her discussions with nurses about tools and techniques of quality assurance. It seems that nurses often start by trying a pre-existing tool which provides them with a good grounding in the principles of quality assurance. Having developed some confidence and broken the ice in the unit, they then move on to producing standards of their own as this is more likely to reflect the needs of the unit as a whole. Most nurses find the exercise of setting standards rewarding work, which helps improve motivation and commitment.

But where does one begin?

In order to lend some kind of structure to standard setting, the RCN
Dynamic Standard Setting approach (Kitson, 1988) is illustrated in Figure
5.1. This system involves a group of ward staff identifying a topic or
problem area for quality improvement, developing the standard and its
associated criteria and employing measurement techniques to determine
how well the standard is met. The group then agrees an appropriate
course of action and evaluates the effect of employing it.

It may be useful to repeat here the definition of 'standard' as given by
the *Chambers Dictionary* (1980) as:

> a basis for measurement, an established or accepted model; a definite
> level of excellence or adequacy required, aimed at or possible.

Greenhalgh and Company (1991) in the section on quality define
'standard' as:

> an agreed level of performance negotiated within available resources.

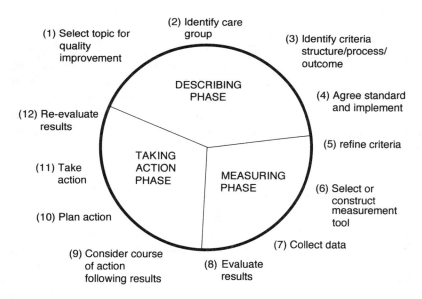

Fig. 5.1   The Quality Assurance Cycle

The RCN dynamic standard setting approach: the Q.A. cycle. Reproduced with
permission of Dr Alison Kitson.

'Criterion' is defined by the *Chambers Dictionary* as:

a means or standard of judging; a test, a rule.

Criteria are the cues or characteristics of a standard that an observer looks for to indicate if a standard is met or not. Criteria are also called 'indicators', 'interpretations' or 'items' in various tools. Standards should be appropriate to the population addressed, observable, achievable, measurable and desirable (RCN, 1986).

Criteria statements should be related to the standard being measured, free of bias, suitable for quantification and statistical treatment and be valid and reliable (Kemp and Richardson, 1990).

An example of a standard statement is taken from *Standards of Care for Cancer Nursing* (RCN Standards of Care Project, 1991):

The nurse ensures that the individual and his family have all the information required to participate in making decisions regarding his disease and treatment.

Standards can originate in two ways according to Donabedian (1966): normative standards derive, in principle, from the source that legitimately sets the standards of knowledge and practice, while empirical standards are derived from actual practice. In practice, nurses developing standards for themselves use a combination of the two.

Standards are usually written on specific topics because they are giving cause for concern or because an innovation is being introduced. It may be useful to use some kind of framework to lend structure to the choice of topics. There is no limit to the number of standards that can be written for a specific topic, but it must be remembered that eventually the quality of care will be measured by evaluating whether or not the standards are met. If there are many standards, this becomes more complex and may need the help of computers and statisticians to aid measurement and the analysis of the results.

When developing standards and criteria, Donabedian (1969) provides a logical and easily applicable approach. Standards and criteria can be divided into structure, process and outcome categories:

Structure   factors in the organization that enable work to be carried out; such as environmental facilities, equipment, staffing, education and management.
Process   the performance of the nurse; the actual care received by the client and work carried out by the nurse.
Outcome   the effect such care has on the patient or client group.

Using the standard statement given above, relating to a client's informational needs, criteria can be developed which reflect these categories. For example, structure criteria might include:

(1)   A nurse is available to assess the informational requirements of the individual.
(2)   The nurse has access to continuing education and support to improve her communication skills.

Process criteria include:

(1)   The nurse makes initial and continuing assessments of the individual's informational requirements and his desire for information.
(2)   The nurse provides individuals or relatives with literature about the disease or treatment when required and is prepared to discuss it in detail with them.

Outcome criteria might include:

(1)   The individual and his family state that they have the information they require regarding diagnosis, treatment and prognosis.
(2)   The individual states he has understood the implications of the treatment options before signing a consent form.

(RCN Standards of Care Project, 1991)

Once the working group has agreed the standards and criteria, these should be submitted for ratification by the unit manager and by the local quality assurance committee, so that coordination of standard setting initiatives can be arranged and to ensure that the standards set are within legal limits and are acceptable to the institution or department.

The list of standard statements and their associated criteria are eventually arranged into some kind of instrument or tool with space for marking by an observer of the quality of care. This can be done in a number of ways and guidance for doing it can be found by looking at the numerous existing tools and associated literature.

The quality assurance cycle is completed by evaluating the results of monitoring quality and then planning and taking action resulting from the exercise. Quality must then be monitored again to ensure that the action taken produces the desired results.

It must be remembered that undertaking a quality assurance exercise can be a threatening experience for nursing staff who are unused to the idea. It is vitally important to minimize this threat so that the results of the quality monitoring can be used to change nursing practice. If the staff are negative about the exercise or feel that it is imposed on them by management, then they may refute the results and resist the ensuing changes. This would make the whole exercise fruitless. There are a variety of ways of ensuring that staff feel positive about quality assurance:

(1) Education: all student nurses should have quality assurance issues introduced to them as a normal part of nursing life. In-service training of qualified staff should help to increase their knowledge of the issues and the problems solved. When quality assurance measures are commencing, all the staff involved should have the opportunity to attend workshops related to the specific method or tool. Each ward or unit involved in a quality-monitoring exercise should be provided with written information about the tool and the method to be used.

(2) Representation: if possible, all grades of staff should be represented on the steering committee to ensure that all feel they have a voice in decision making. Representatives from the units involved should participate in developing any new tools or methods for quality measurement.

(3) Respected observers: when undertaking a monitoring exercise, the observers should be individuals whose judgement and clinical knowledge is respected by the ward staff. They may even be members of staff. This should increase the chances of staff agreeing with results.

(4) Feedback: results of the exercise should be fed back to individual units as quickly as possible and anonymity should be ensured. It is important that staff do not view quality monitoring as a way of developing a league chart of units or wards, but as a way of improving or maintaining their own standards. No cross-ward or cross-unit comparisons should be made, but only changes that occur on one unit with the lapse of time. Ward staff should be made to feel that they 'own' the results of the monitoring exercise and can use them as they wish. Incentives could be offered to encourage improvements in standards.

(5) Involvement: all staff should be given ample opportunity to become involved at all stages.

These guidelines for the setting of standards and criteria and for quality assurance generally are not to be seen as hard-and-fast rules, but are presented here as possibilities for working groups to look at. They also serve as an introduction to the terminology involved. It is hoped that this chapter has addressed some of the issues related to quality assurance and provided enough information and practical tips to enable nurses at relatively junior levels to feel they might want to, and that they could, participate in, or even initiate, quality assurance measures within their own units.

References

Ball, J.A., Goldstone, L.A. & Collier, M.M. (1984) *Criteria for Care – The manual of the North West nurse staffing levels project* Newcastle upon Tyne Polytechnic Products Ltd, Newcastle upon Tyne.

Barnett, D. and Wainwright, P. (1987) Between two tools *Senior Nurse* **6**(4), 40–2.

Brittle, J. & Marsh, J. (1986) Definition of Measurement? *Nursing Times* Nov 5, 36–7.

Close, A. (1990) Tools and Techniques *Nursing Standard* **5**(9), Quality Assurance Supplement.

Dunn, C. (1990) Who Cares? *Nursing Standard* **5**(9) Quality Assurance Supplement, 6.

Goldstone, L.A., Ball, J.A. & Collier, M.M. (1984) *Monitor – An Index of the Quality of Nursing Care for Acute Medical and Surgical Wards* Newcastle upon Tyne Polytechnical Products Ltd., Newcastle upon Tyne, England.

Greenhalgh and Company in conjunction with a Five Regional Consortium (1991) *Using Information in Managing the Nursing Resource*, Crown Copyright.

Hegyvary, S.T. & Haussmann, R.K.D. (1975) Monitoring Nursing Care Quality. *Journal of Nursing Administration*, June 17–26.

Kemp, N. and Richardson, E. (1990) *Quality Assurance in Nursing Practice.* Butterworth-Heinemann Ltd, Oxford.

Little, W., Fowler, H.W. and Coulson, J. (1983) *The Shorter Oxford English Dictionary* 3rd edition, Oxford University Press, Oxford.

MacDonald, A.M. (ed.) (1980) *Chambers Dictionary* Chambers, London.

NHS Management Executive (May 1991) *Framework of audit for nursing services.*

PA Consulting Services Ltd., (1987) *Nursing Quality Measurement Scale* PA Consulting Services Ltd. Knightsbridge, London.

Phaneuf, M. (1976) *The Nursing Audit – Self Regulation in Nursing Practice* 2nd edn, Appleton–Century–Croft, New York.

Report of an inquiry into the management of the health service to the Secretary of State (1983) (*The Griffiths Report*). HMSO, London.

RCN Standards of Care Project (1986) *Check list on how to write standards of nursing care*, Royal College of Nursing, London.

RCN Standards of Care Project (1991) *Standards of Care for Cancer Nursing*, Royal College of Nursing, London.

UKCC (1984) *Code of Professional Conduct for the Nurse, Midwife and Health Visitor* UKCC, London.

Wandelt, M.A. & Ager, J.W. (1974) *Quality Patient Care Scale* Appleton–Century–Croft, New York.

Whelan, J. (1987) Using Monitor – Observer Bias *Senior Nurse* **7**(6), 8–10.

World Health Organization (March, 1986), *Nursing/Midwifery in Europe*, WHO Regional Unit for Europe.

Recommended Reading

Pearson, A. (1987) *Nursing quality measurement: quality assurance methods for peer review*, John Wiley and Sons, Chichester.

Wilson, C. (1987) *Hospital Wide Quality Assurance*, W.B. Saunders, Canada.

Chapter 6
Day-to-day organization in the ward

Ward sisters or charge nurses would wish to make the best use of the resources at their disposal so that wards run efficiently and smoothly. Their main resources are staff members, time, equipment and the ward itself, and these should be organized and used effectively if patients are to receive a high level of nursing care and if nurses are to obtain satisfaction from their work (Fig. 6.1). Patients and their relatives rely on that organizing ability for satisfactory nursing care.

An individualized approach to patients is accepted as being the best way to nurse patients, and therefore the ward must be organized so that the nurses are able to achieve this – as will be discussed in this chapter.

Flexibility is most important when planning the patients' day or organizing the nursing team. The sister or charge nurse who has a rigid attitude to the organization of the ward and function of the nursing

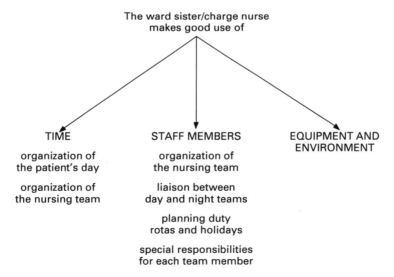

Fig. 6.1   Effective use of the resources within the ward.

team will demonstrate a rigid approach to all aspects of patient care. Care in the ward will become indiscriminate rather than thoughtful and imaginative, and nurses are discouraged from treating patients as people and are not able to plan to meet individual needs.

The patients' day and organization of patient care within the ward vary from one speciality to another. This is another reason for a flexible approach. What is right for a neurosurgical ward will not necessarily be right for an ophthalmic ward. Each ward must be critically appraised.

Organization of the patients' day

A plan for the organization of the patients' day is necessary so that staff and patients feel secure, although this may be argued against by some. Traditionally, certain procedures have been carried out and completed by a certain time: for example, all patients bathed in the morning, all dressings renewed in the morning, the night nurse administers many of the daily drugs. A more flexible day, but retaining some routine to give security to both patients and staff so that everyone knows what is likely to happen at a given time, leads to a happier ward. It is important that the day is planned around the patients' needs rather than the needs of the nurses or doctors.

When looking at the patients' day many factors must be borne in mind:

(1) The hospital's operational policy – can this be adapted in a flexible way?
(2) The services that are provided at set times by other departments, e.g. patients' meals, staff meals, domestic services.
(3) Input of other personnel having direct patient contact, e.g. phlebotomist, physiotherapist, doctors.
(4) Time of drug rounds: can they be altered if this will improve the ward organization? Is it necessary to do a drug round or could the nurse responsible for care give drugs to her patients as needed?
(5) Patient turnover: in a ward with high patient turnover the priorities in care will be the admission of, caring for and discharge of patients rather than the routine of meal times and drug times. For longer stay settings, a more organized patient day becomes possible.

It may not be possible to alter some established practices because of the effect on other disciplines, for example, meal times. After considering the more routine aspects of the patients' stay in hospital, established operational practices can provide a framework on which to base the ward pattern of the patients' day, allowing a more individual approach to each patient. Also, now that all disciplines are becoming increasingly aware of the need to continually aim to improve the quality of patient care, it is easier to change established practices.

Each nurse should be encouraged to plan her or his work for the whole shift, emphasis being made on getting the priorities for patient care correct. This should get rid of the mythical 12 noon deadline by which time nurses feel they must have completed all their work. Priority should be given to the patients' general comfort and prevention of pressure sores, to required fluid intake, preparation for special tests, preparation for discharge, and listening to patients, rather than bathing, bedmaking, and 'getting everything done'. The sister or charge nurse must continue to reinforce this philosophy to the permanent team members and to those arriving new to the ward. The staff will be helped if the sister or charge nurse:

- Delegates with authority but remains accountable
- Allows the nurses time to plan their work
- Does not expect everything to be completed by lunchtime
- Encourages each shift to work with the next during overlap periods
- Communicates effectively and allows time for the nurses to report back, especially at the change-over of each shift and at staff meal times.
- Involves the nurse responsible for the patient in any decision-making
- Ensures that the ward is adequately covered at all times, especially during meal breaks, i.e., if two registered general nurses are on duty they go to separate meal breaks.

Organization of nursing care

Virginia Henderson (1968) stated that 'the unique function of the nurse is to assist the individual, sick or well, in the performance of those activities of daily living which he or she would normally perform unaided, to help him or her to recover health or, if that is impossible, to help him or her towards a peaceful death'. The nurse's job ranges from maintaining the patient's quality of self-care to meeting the needs of the totally dependent patient.

Each person has certain needs which must be fulfilled, both in health and in sickness. These needs can be described in several ways. Maslow (1968) described them as a hierarchy of needs, with the basic needs being fulfilled before the higher needs can be considered (Fig. 6.2). As each need is satisfied the next one takes its place.

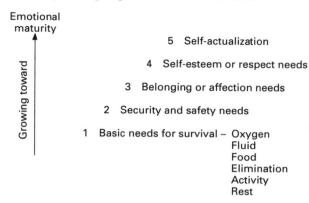

Fig. 6.2 Maslow's hierarchy of needs.

Henderson (1968), when considering the patient, stated that needs are the foundation of nursing care.

The art of being a good ward sister or charge nurse is in enabling the nursing team to meet the patients' needs efficiently and effectively. This takes organization! It is useful to have a model or framework or guidelines on which to base decisions regarding the organization of nursing care, both on a day-to-day basis as well as in the longer term.

Models of nursing

There are several models or theories of nursing which can be used as tools for studying and understanding nursing, assessing patients' needs and planning nursing action. Some are practical but others are more abstract and may be difficult to apply within a ward. The aim of each is to focus on the patient as an individual with nursing rather than medical needs and problems, although the two cannot be divorced. We will mention here a few of the more well-known models so that the reader can read more widely about a particular model of her or his choice.

Roper's activities of living model

This looks at the person in terms of activities of daily living able to be performed. Nursing intervention is indicated when the patient is unable to perform these.

Activities of daily living:

(1) Maintaining a safe environment
(2) Communicating

(3)   Breathing
(4)   Eating and drinking
(5)   Eliminating
(6)   Personal cleansing and dressing
(7)   Controlling body temperature
(8)   Mobilizing
(9)   Working and playing
(10) Expressing sexuality
(11) Sleeping
(12) Dying.

Henderson's model of nursing

This model is based on the individual's fundamental human needs, and nursing care is indicated when a patient is unable to meet these needs. The patient's needs are to:

(1)   Breathe normally
(2)   Eat and drink adequately
(3)   Eliminate by all avenues of elimination
(4)   Move and maintain desired position
(5)   Sleep and rest
(6)   Dress and undress and select suitable clothing
(7)   Maintain body temperature – adjust clothing or modify environment
(8)   Keep body clean, well groomed and protect the integument
(9)   Avoid dangers in the environment
(10) Communicate and express emotions, needs and fears
(11) Worship according to faith or conform to concept of right and wrong
(12) Work at something which gives a sense of accomplishment
(13) Play and participate in recreation
(14) Learn, discover or satisfy the curiosity.

Orem's self-care model

Orem sees a balance between an individual's self-care abilities and present demands being made on him or her. Nursing care is indicated when this balance is lost, and as the patient becomes less able to help him or herself because of disability or ill-health, the nursing input increases to enable the patient to meet his or her needs.

Roy's adaptation model

Nursing problems arise when there are disturbances of the physiological, psychological or sociological systems affecting the behaviour of the individual. Nursing intervention is indicated so that the patient can be helped to adapt to these changes, enabling him or her to cope. The patient's energy can then be channelled into promoting well-being.

There are other models (e.g. Neuman's and Roger's), but those cited here are the most common. The majority of the models have been developed in America – the exception being Roper's. The choice of which model to use may be a difficult one and may depend on the type of patient in the ward. For example, it might not be appropriate to use Orem's Self-Care Model in a ward where nearly all the patients are highly dependent (as in Intensive Care) where the aim of care may not be self-care, but merely the return to a state of less dependence on medical and nursing support, and transfer to a unit where rehabilitation can commence. Some models may be particularly appropriate for specific settings, such as the use of Roy's adaptation model in psychiatric settings.

Whichever model, or models, or mixture of models, is chosen it should be understood and agreed by all the nursing staff on the ward and incorporated into a statement of the ward philosophy of care. This forms the basis for the systematic application of the nursing process.

The nursing process

The aim of good nursing care is to build up a picture of the patient as a unique person within a family and community, and then to decide the best way to help the patient. This will include both the care required to meet the patients' needs and resolve the nursing problems, and the goals to be attained. Care is based on the patients' individual needs – physical, emotional, psychological, social and spiritual – as well as on those related to the medical reason for being in hospital.

If patients' needs are not met, nursing problems are likely to occur. The most effective method of assessing and meeting patients' needs is by using the concept of the nursing process, a systematic approach to assessing patients' needs, planning and delivering care, which provides a framework for an individual nursing approach. It is essential that nurses are allocated to patients as opposed to tasks if these concepts are to be effective. The patients must be involved in any decision-making related to their care, and the nurses must have a desire to encourage independence of function as fully as possible. The nursing care for each patient must be individually planned, continuous, and consistent.

The stages of the nursing process are: assessment of the patients and their nursing problems and needs; planning the nursing care; implementing the nursing care plan, and then evaluating the effectiveness of the care given, and adjusting the plan accordingly.

If the concept of the nursing process is followed, it should achieve:

- An individual approach to each patient
- A systematic method of determining patients' needs and problems
- Systematic planning of care which is written down and describes how the needs are to be met and the problems solved
- Continuity of care
- Continuous updating of care
- Written, permanent nursing records
- Evaluation of care
- A tool for monitoring the quality of care
- A record of information for research purposes.

It must be emphasized that the interpretation of the nursing process will vary from ward to ward. It is, however, concerned with the welfare of the patients and will always involve the patients and their families in the decision-making. All the stages are recorded to give a permanent record of needs and problems, action to be taken, goals to be achieved, and eventual outcome.

Assessment

Assessment of each patient is made on admission and involves:

(1) Obtaining information from the patient or relatives
(2) Observation of the patient's physical and emotional state
(3) Sifting the information and identifying the needs and problems

Obtaining information

Before care can be planned the nurse must carefully observe the patient and obtain all relevant information. The success or otherwise of obtaining information will depend on the building up of a relationship between the nurse and the patient. It is important to decide beforehand what information is being sought as some information will be common to all nursing situations. Other information will be determined by the individual patient's needs. 'Individual' is emphasized to remind the nurse seeking the information that this is to be a part of the 'individualized approach'. In particular, when obtaining information from a patient the nurse must be close enough to the patient to observe the way in which a question is answered, the slightest worry or concern on the face of the patient that contradicts a positive reply, or the gestures that indicate tension when the exact opposite has been stated.

The depth of information required will be determined by the patient's length of stay in hospital, the reason for admission and degree of dependence on the nursing team. Knowledge of food likes and dislikes is not as important for patients admitted for a series of investigations, who are able to attend to their own needs. If, however, a patient has a communication problem such as aphasia following a stroke, it is vital that food likes and dislikes are discovered. If a patient is fully ambulant, noting the normal degree of mobility is not as important as with an elderly patient following a fractured femur or stroke.

Information is obtained from the patient or, if appropriate, a close relative or friend. The information being sought is private and privileged and should be obtained in a manner appropriate to confidence.

The doctors' case notes are also a source of information and, if used properly, will avoid the patient being subjected to the same questions more than once.

In some instances, information will be obtained from other health care workers such as the general practitioner, social worker, district nurse or health visitor if these people have been involved in the care of the patient prior to admission.

All the information obtained relating to the patient's preadmission state is usually referred to as the nursing history. It may take one of several styles such as a detailed questionnaire, a checklist or an interview guide. The questions asked reflect the model of nursing used on the unit, but all are aimed at building up a full picture of the patient, his background, family, home circumstances and problems. In addition, there may be questions that relate to the patient's illness and hospitalization, or which are specific to the unit.

For example, a woman being admitted for a hip replacement, should be asked details of the geography of her home, noting things like the position of the toilets, the presence of stairs, and the amount of help she might have available. These things help in planning for her discharge.

When a child is admitted, the name by which he would like to be called should be noted (as it should for any patient!) as well as the names and descriptions of any toys he has brought with him.

All the information need not be obtained at the time of admission, but can be added to day-by-day. This will depend on the patient's immediate needs and the pressures within the ward at the time. The closer the relationship between patient and nurse, the better the opportunity for the nurse to obtain the required information. The nurse must become involved and must decide, with guidance from the sister or charge nurse, the information required immediately and that which is best left until later.

Once a rapport has been established the nurse will need to explore unobtrusively the patients' feelings about being ill and their reaction to being in hospital, as well as the nurse's own feelings towards caring for each patient.

Observation of the patient

As well as gathering information from the patient or the relatives, the nurse must also observe the patient's general appearance, state of the mouth and skin, any abnormalities, mannerisms, physical signs of fatigue, emotions, anxieties and fears.

Such a baseline observation is very important as it provides the basis for the identification and monitoring of problems throughout the patient's stay in hospital. The structure of the observations will vary depending on the model for care used on the ward and what the patient's admitting problems are. Some of the commonly used guidelines are the activities of daily living described by Roper (1982).

Communications skills are obviously extremely important and the art of interviewing and listening to the patient develops with experience. Junior nurses will need help and guidance from the ward sister or charge nurse, who must convey to the nurses the importance of sitting and talking to, and listening to their patients, stressing that sitting and listening does not imply idleness. The information may be obtained and recorded on a structured form, or used to write a comprehensive summary of observations.

Sifting the information and identifying needs and problems

Having obtained the information the nurse then sifts it and identifies needs and problems. This is followed by assessing priorities, setting nursing goals and making plans to meet the patient's needs, remembering that basic needs will exist for any patient in any setting, regardless of the clinical diagnosis. However, some patients may be able to meet most of their own physical needs at most times, provided help is readily available if required.

The nurse must help patients meet their emotional needs such as coming to terms with their illness or disability. It must never be assumed that patients are able to attend to their own basic needs just because they are mobile. They may be physically capable but sometimes it is not only a measurement of physical capacity that is necessary. The less obvious needs may seemingly be met but in fact are not so, nothing must ever be taken for granted or assumed. There has to be a balance between the needs the patient is able to meet alone and those which the nurse must meet, and it is important that the nurse develops a sensitivity to recognize when intervention is necessary.

The patients' nursing problems may be immediate or potential.

Immediate problems

Problems which must be dealt with at the time of admission are *immediate*. Some of the immediate problems will need urgent nursing intervention. For example, an immediate problem for an unconscious patient will be the maintenance of a clear airway, and the goal is to enable the patient to maintain adequate respiration.

Potential problems

Potential problems are those which may develop in the future. These can be anticipated and therefore prevented or minimized in many instances; they emphasize the need to plan ahead. For example, an elderly lady who has had a cerebrovascular accident leaving her with a hemiparesis, falls and fractures her femur. Because of reduced mobility she is at risk of developing pressure sores, deep vein thrombosis and hypostatic pneumonia unless these potential problems are anticipated and the appropriate nursing care planned.

Veiled problems

Some problems are more obvious than others. Those illustrated are obvious immediate and potential problems. Others are more difficult to ascertain, as patients respond in different ways to their illness, its treatment, hospitalization and their own social and economic environment.

Mrs Hawthorn is 82 years old, and lives alone in poor accommodation in a condemned area of the inner city. Following admission to hospital, the nurses, Mrs Hawthorn's relatives and social worker feel strongly that she must be rehoused. Mrs Hawthorn is very independent and is adamant that she wants to go back to her own home where she is quite happy and content. For the patient there is no problem, but the hospital staff and relatives had assumed a problem existed.

The nurse must talk to the patient to find out how the patient views the situation and to involve the patients in all decision-making which affects them.

Apparent problems are not always the real problems. Needs and problems can be difficult to identify and can therefore be neglected. For example, if a nurse or doctor is admitted to hospital it is often assumed that their need for safety and security has been met in that they know how to act as a patient, they understand what is going to happen to them and so they feel secure. However, as with any other patient they may have a fear of hospitals, surgery, anaesthesia or injections and their need for security and reassurance is just as real as with any other patient. All patients need help from the nurses in coming to terms with the position they find themselves in.

If information is not sifted and patients' needs are not assessed, care becomes routine and indiscriminate – the same for each patient, no matter what that patient's individual needs are. The ward routine becomes all important, and the needs of the ward are met rather than those of the patient.

Mrs Lime was a meticulous 35-year-old mother of two, with an outgoing personality. She attended the outpatient clinic one afternoon, and before leaving home for the hospital she had a shower. That night she developed a pulmonary embolus, became critically ill and was admitted to hospital. An intravenous infusion was commenced, she needed continuous oxygen therapy and regular analgesia. Immediately after breakfast the following morning she was given a complete bedbath which made her feel worse rather than more comfortable. Mrs Lime thought this most unnecessary as she had had a shower the previous day, but no one had bothered to assess her needs properly, or to involve her in the decision.

Planning

As soon as needs and problems have been determined care is planned to meet the assessed needs and to avoid potential problems. This becomes possible by planning ahead.

Planning is easier if done systematically, by asking:

- What is to be done?
- What are the problems?
- What are we trying to achieve?
- Why is it to be done?
- When is it to be done?
- Where is it to be done?

If planning is done in a systematic way valuable nursing time will be saved. If recorded, the planning can be shared with all those who are involved in the care of the patient. It will also remove any discrepancy between the care the sister or charge nurse thinks is being given and that which is given. When planning care, the nurse must remember:

(1) Constraints within the system that are not possible to alter, for example, set meal times.
(2) Professional resources and equipment. It is important to match the level of care to be given against the resources available.
(3) The patients' ability to help themselves and the need to encourage self-care, while ensuring that the nurse allocated to care for the patient continues to observe the patient and provide support as indicated.
(4) The need to involve the patients in decision-making which relates to themselves, and possibly the need to involve their relatives and other disciplines.
(5) Respect for individual idiosyncrasies on the part of the patient.
(6) The need to encourage independence and individuality, for example, the wearing of day clothes rather than dressing gowns and pyjamas and freedom of mobility such as being able to go to the hospital shop or into the grounds, as long as the ward staff know where to find the patient.

Care must always be planned to meet the needs of the patients, and this responsibility should be that of a trained nurse who should have developed interpersonal skills and is able to assess and interpret the facts and who also has the necessary clinical knowledge and expertise. A senior student nurse should also be capable of planning care effectively as long as guidance is given by the trained nurse.

Care is planned giving first consideration to priorities, but some priorities are more obvious than others. For example, the maintenance of the airway before cleanliness is obvious, but sleep and rest before cleanliness is less obvious to some nurses.

Involvement of the patient in decision-making is essential for the patient's comfort when in hospital. A good example is the daily ritual of bathing that still occurs in some hospitals. Some patients prefer to bath once a week or less. Therefore, unless there is a specific nursing or medical reason for more frequent baths, as with the incontinent patient or the patient who has been prescribed medicated baths, discussion with the patient is vital. It might be that the patient is frightened to bath at home but with help would prefer to bath more frequently. On the other hand, the patient may prefer to continue with weekly baths. Some patients may like to have their bath in the evening rather than the usual morning or afternoon. Some patients prefer a shower and vice versa; therefore, again, discussion with the patient is essential.

> Mr Berry was an elderly man who had had treatment for cardiac failure and was waiting for a place in a social care home. Despite his protests he was put in the bath every day. The nurses told him that it was sister's wish. Much distress to the patient could have been avoided if the sister, with the nurse, had discussed his normal bathing pattern with him.

> Mrs Pine has lobar pneumonia and initially is to rest in bed. She is obese. When toilet needs are considered the nurse planning her care discusses with Mrs Pine whether she prefers to use a bedpan, commode at the bedside or to be taken to the toilet in a wheelchair. She is reassured that, whatever method she prefers and is the least exhausting, there will be a nurse to give her all the assistance she requires.

Patients must also be actively involved in decision-making related to the time of day when they would prefer to sit out of bed, if they are allowed out of bed for a limited time. One patient may prefer to sit out when the family visits, but another might choose to sit out of bed for meals.

When planning care, it may be necessary for the nurse to seek further information or suggestions from other sources, such as nurse specialists, physiotherapists, doctors or pharmacists, or from books or journal articles. In this way the clinical nurse can ensure her knowledge base is updated and she can implement research findings in patient care.

When planning nursing care the objectives should be stated positively, so that there are goals to aim for. This is illustrated in the following examples.

Example 1

An unconscious patient is admitted to the ward, following an overdose of drugs.

Nursing problem	Nursing goal	Nursing care plan or nursing prescription
Unconscious and unable to breathe normaly	Maintain a clear airway at all times	Remove dentures; nurse in semi-prone position

Example 2

An elderly lady, following a cerebrovascular accident which had left her with a right hemiparesis, falls and fractures her right leg.

Nursing problem	Nursing goal	Nursing care plan or nursing prescription
Reduced mobility At risk of developing:		
Pressure sores	Maintain skin in healthy and intact condition	Keep skin clean and dry; ease position 1–2 hourly; nurse on full-length sheepskin; assess skin integrity twice daily.
Deep vein thrombosis	Maintain good venous return	Encourage to move toes hourly; encourage to move left leg 2-hourly, passive movements of toes of right foot by nurse 2-hourly; refer to physiotherapist; teach patient and observe for signs of thrombosis.
Hypostatic pneumonia	Maintain full inspiration and expiration	Encourage to take deep breaths every hour; observe for signs of pneumonia – i.e. raised temperature, pulse and respiratory rate.

Implementation of the care plan

The nurse carries out the prescribed care during her or his span of duty. The method of ward organization and the allocation of nurses to their patients will depend on several factors. However, to implement the care plan effectively the nurse must have responsibility for the total care of that patient.

If a support worker is given the responsibility of caring for a small group of patients such as preconvalescent patients, a care plan, formulated by a trained nurse, will be available. The support worker will also be supervised by a trained nurse for the whole of the duty span.

The nurses delegated to the care of specific patients are held accountable for the care given. They are responsible for giving a clear verbal report, reviewing and updating the care plan and writing the nursing records accurately and completely. The sister or charge nurse may consider it necessary to guide a nurse, especially a trainee, and should be available to give advice if needed.

Records must be completed in detail in order that a proper picture of the patient's stay in hospital is always available. An example of a very poor entry in the nursing records is:

2.00 p.m.	Fair morning – remains lethargic.
	For home tomorrow.
	Temp. 2 p.m. 38°
6.00 a.m.	Satisfactory night. Slept well.
11.00 a.m.	Discharged home. For admission
	to hospital B on Tuesday.

The patient's wife complained later that her husband had had a high temperature when he arrived home from Hospital A. The nursing records were consulted but were of no value at all, even though it was later discovered that he had, in fact, been sent home whilst his temperature was elevated, but the doctor had been consulted prior to his discharge and had felt that the patient was fit enough to go home. This information should have been recorded in the nursing report.

If nursing records are inadequate continuity of care is at risk. This is because nurses are working fewer hours, more part-time nurses are employed, more health care professionals including more medical specialists are involved in the patient's care and treatment. The nursing records are legal documents and if a complaint is made against the hospital it is vital that the necessary information is available in the nursing report.

Evaluation of care

Evaluation of care can be difficult, but if care is not evaluated nursing standards will never be improved. Nurses have been reluctant to look critically at standards of care and methods of ward organization in the past and this has led to many facets of care becoming rigid routines rather than individualized care. Nurses should learn from their mistakes if nursing care is to be improved.

Evaluation can be threatening, but if carried out positively and objectively it will result in an improvement in care, ward organization and teaching. Objectivity is needed when evaluating care, and evaluation is often best achieved by group discussion with the whole nursing team present. The involvement of the patient and the patient's family is also necessary.

Evaluation takes place constantly. To help evaluate care certain questions may be asked, such as:

● Could care for this patient be more effective?
● Have the nursing problems been correctly assessed or only the apparent problems taken into consideration?

- Are the goals the right goals?
- Is the prescribed nursing care being effective?
- Is the care being given? For example, if the prescribed care is to turn the patient every two hours, is this being done?
- Is the care realistic?
- Is the nurse's response the right response?
- What changes have occurred which necessitate reassessment of needs and care?
- What has been the response of the patient and his family to the care the patient has received?

Returning to the original example, evaluation could be as follows:

Nursing problem 12th May	Nursing Goal	Nursing care plan or nursing prescription	Evaluation
Reduced mobility At risk of developing Pressure sores	Maintain skin in healthy and intact condition	Keep skin clean and dry, ease position 1–2 hourly, nurse on full-length sheepskin	15th May Skin over buttocks red but intact

As a result of the evaluation, the prescribed care may need to change. The frequency with which evaluation is carried out will vary from patient to patient and depend on the nature of the problem. The evaluation of the care given to a patient in an intensive care unit will probably be carried out several times over the period of a day. On the other hand, the evaluation of the care of a patient who is being rehabilitated following a cerebrovascular accident will probably only be of value if carried out weekly or even fortnightly.

Evaluation is based to a large extent on the observation of the patient – the patient's general condition, progress and response to care. Such things as state of the skin or mouth, level of mobility and independence will be considered, and will relate to the expected progress for that patient. The way the patient feels and whether he or she considers that the rate of progress has come up to expectations will also help the nurse to evaluate care.

Following the evaluation of the care prescribed, the nursing care plan will often need to be reviewed and adjusted or completely changed. The goals may need to be altered if it is felt that they are unrealistic.

During evaluation, it is also necessary to discover any other reason why care has not been carried out as planned. This will assist in reviewing the method of ward organization which should also be under constant assessment. It may be found that there was:

- Insufficient information obtained at the assessment stage
- A lack of necessary information
- Failure to record important information
- Failure to communicate with patient or relatives
- Failure to consider the importance of the input of the family
- Lack of knowledge on the part of the nurse concerned
- Lack of initiative by the nurse concerned
- Lack of knowledge and understanding of the nursing process
- Breakdown in good relationships between members of staff because of wrong attitudes
- Resistance to change
- Inadequate recording of information obtained and care to be given
- Non-adherence to nursing principles and hospital policies.

Sisters and charge nurses and their staff should adopt a flexible attitude to the nursing process. If the principles (Table 6.1) are accepted the process can be adapted to any ward. It must be remembered, however, that what works well in one ward will not necessarily work in another. If it is adopted and adjusted to the ward it will not work effectively straightaway but time must be allowed for experimentation and re-appraisal after first considering the practical implications.

The nursing process enables the registered nurse to set individual standards for patients, and when evaluating care the outcome of the care given is compared with the aims of care set. If care is properly evaluated this should lead to an improvement in the standard of care given.

Organizing patient care

Although most hospitals have now adopted the use of individualized patient care, some nurses still feel that this has been thrust upon them without much explanation, and others still maintain a preference for task allocation. For their benefit, it is worth reviewing the advantages and disadvantages of both methods of organizing patient care. These are not based entirely on research findings or literature, but on personal experience and observation, and from talking to all grades of staff using the various systems.

Table 6.1   A summary of the steps of the nursing process.

IDENTIFY AND ASSESS patient's needs and problems by
   observing
   talking
   listening
   negotiating
PLAN to meet the needs and solve and anticipate problems by
   discussion with the patient
                the patient's family
                the nursing team
                health care workers
   documentation
IMPLEMENT THE PLAN
EVALUATE THE CARE GIVEN by
   observation
   discussion with the patient
                the patient's family
                the nursing team

Individualized care

Individualized care is defined as caring for the patient's entire needs as a planned and complete procedure by one or more nurses. All the patient's needs are met as far as possible – i.e. emotional, spiritual, physical, educational, environmental, social, economic and rehabilitative needs. The patient is recognized as a member of a family and of the community, and care will include helping the patient and the patient's family to adjust to the new situation.

Care will involve communication with the patient and his family as well as with other health care professionals – both within the hospital and in the community.

Individualized care is planned with the patient's individual needs – along with the needs of the other patients for whom the nurse is responsible – being taken into account. One patient may benefit by being allowed to rest for as long as possible, while another may need frequent stimulation.

Advantages of individualized care

General

(1)   The emphasis is put back on basic as opposed to technical care for all grades of nurse. 'It is wrong to assume that basic nursing is easy and can be relegated to learners or untrained staff, while technical

care is difficult and the preserve of the trained nurse' (McFarlane 1977).

(2)   Improved nursing documentation is encouraged and the nursing process can readily be applied.

(3)   There is improved communication within the ward, with a more integrated system of nursing care.

(4)   Team morale is high – work is more varied and interesting, with more responsibility and experience for all nurses in all aspects of patient care, leading to greater job satisfaction. People with job satisfaction give better patient care.

(5)   Sickness and absenteeism are reduced.

(6)   Time is used more effectively.

To the patients

(1)   The nurse/patient relationship is improved. As there is closer contact with fewer nurses a better rapport is achieved.

(2)   The patients are able to obtain information tailored to their needs.

(3)   Emphasis is on the patients' needs rather than on the needs of the ward so patients' individual needs become more apparent.

(4)   Nursing care is planned systematically and individually and is not fragmented.

(5)   The ward routine is arranged round the patients leaving them more time to rest.

(6)   The patients are involved, along with their family if indicated, in the planning and delivery of their care.

(7)   Fear of hospitals is reduced if a personal approach is made to the patients on admission.

To the nurses

(1)   The nurses feel more involved and have a feeling of belonging to the ward.

(2)   The nurses get to know the patients better as they are involved with fewer patients, and are in a better position to observe, assess and meet the needs of each patient.

(3)   The nurses in training have more contact with other nurses, doctors and health care workers as they need to communicate with these personnel about their patients.

(4)   The nurses are able to develop their own individuality for caring.

(5)   The nurses feel more secure and gain confidence – they know their patients and this gives confidence in relating to them and caring for them. This also gives an improved learning situation,

with an opportunity for each nursing action to be clearly understood.

(6) The nurses have more responsibility but are aware that support and guidance is at hand.

(7) Trained nurses become more caring and responsive to the needs of the patient as they are accountable for the care they give.

(8) Part-time trained nurses are used more efficiently.

(9) Training for leadership is enhanced.

(10) The nurses develop expertise in written and verbal communication.

(11) Experience during nurse training becomes more varied and meaningful.

To the ward sisters and charge nurses

(1) They are in a supervisory role, with time to give support, guidance and advice, enabling others to draw on their wealth of experience. The ward is more efficiently supervised.

(2) There is time to teach patients, their relatives and staff.

(3) There is an awareness of who is directly responsible and therefore accountable for all aspects of care.

(4) They know who to approach concerning changes in treatment, or if information is required about a patient.

(5) They are able to apply management techniques such as communication, leadership, estimation of resources, delegation.

(6) They have more time to know what is happening over-all, while they must direct the doctor to the nurse responsible for each patient.

Disadvantages and difficulties of individualized patient care

General

(1) There must be coordination of effort by the permanent trained staff of the ward so that the same system of organization is followed by whoever is in charge of the ward. Team morale must be high and team members loyal to each other.

(2) Support must be seen to be given by nursing management.

(3) Resistance from doctors: nurses are encouraged to act and think independently, developing their own autonomy, and this can be seen as a threat. The doctors may find it difficult to relate to anyone other than the ward sister or charge nurse.

(4) There may be difficulty in evenly distributing the workload.

(5) There may be insufficient room for storage of the small amount of extra equipment which may be required.

(6) There may be a breakdown during crises or stressful situations, especially if there is also a reduction in staffing levels, with a tendency to revert back to job allocation.

(7) To be effective, patient allocation requires a certain number of nurses – this will depend on the type and size of ward.

(8) Communications may fail, especially if set times for handovers are not enforced.

(9) Disorganization may occur during the overlap of shifts.

To the patients

(1) They may feel isolated if all the nurses on the ward are not involved in their care.

To the nurses

(1) If short of trained nurses, there may be lack of supervision for the nurses in training.

(2) The learners may not be aware of their own limitations and may not seek advice when needed.

(3) Some nurses may tend to isolate themselves from the rest of the ward and become unaware of the needs and problems of the other patients.

(4) Some nurses may be unable to grasp the principles if they have been used to task-assignment in other areas.

(5) Some nurses may feel unable to use their initiative even when given the opportunity to do so.

To the ward sisters or charge nurses

(1) They may feel threatened because they have to hand over the responsibility for the delivery of care to the nurses.

(2) There are no written checklists of tasks completed.

(3) There may be a fear of delegating as they feel that they will not know what is happening, or are unsure of the capabilities of the nurses.

Task or job assignment

Task assignment is the allocation of jobs to individuals by the person in charge of the ward. These are to be performed as isolated activities which, when combined with the work of the other individual nurses, provide the patients with all the care they need. Nurses are given responsibilities which are appropriate to their grade and part-time nurses are often used as 'extras' to be called upon by whoever needs them.

With this type of ward organization, each nurse has a list of tasks to perform which may include every patient on the ward, with no responsibility to do other than the tasks delegated to them. Sometimes the nurses are left to muddle through, being expected to work down their task list without guidance or support. With job allocation there is a lack of individual care planning – the care of each patient being fitted into the ward routine, which is usually rigid. There is a hierarchy of care: technical care being delegated upwards, and nursing care downwards. The opportunity for observing the patient and developing a rapport is given to the most inexperienced and least trained nurses as this usually occurs when basic nursing care is being given. Job satisfaction is achieved by only a few.

Physically, the patient may have received excellent care by each nurse playing a small part. However, no one has attended to the whole patient who is then rarely seen as an individual in his or her own right. The nurse–patient relationship is fragmented.

Task or job assignment has far less to offer as a method of organizing patient care and is *not recommended.*

The nursing team

The nursing team may be organized in a number of ways. Many factors will influence the type of organization which the sister or charge nurse chooses. The most important are:

- Staffing levels
- Skill mix
- Ward design, for example, Nightingale, race-track, small rooms
- Patient turnover
- Type of patients nursed in the ward.

Each ward sister or charge nurse must adapt to her or his own situation, bearing in mind the aims for the nursing team:

(1) To give a high standard of patient care.
(2) To nurse patients as individuals and meet their needs.
(3) To ensure that each member of the nursing team obtains job satisfaction.

The ward sister or charge nurse may choose one method of organizing the nursing team, and later modify it or change it altogether, until she or he finds a system which suits her or his particular ward. This must be done in full consultation with the other members of the ward team, of course. As ideas are suggested by others in the future she or he may re-appraise the system. It is important that the sister or charge nurse is prepared to look at new methods of organization and patient care – always being open to ideas and suggestions for improvement.

The established methods of organizing care so that individual patient's needs are met are:

- Team nursing
- Patient allocation or case assignment
- Primary nursing.

It is possible to combine various aspects of these three methods of care, and also to change from one to another as the ward sister or charge nurse becomes more experienced and confident, provided this change is planned.

Team nursing

With team nursing the nursing staff is divided into teams, usually two or three per ward, with each team being led by an experienced nurse. Thus, the patient is cared for by a smaller number of nurses with whom he or she can build a relationship and to whom the patient's needs are more apparent.

The ward is divided into two or more areas, with each group of patients in proximity. The layout of the ward will determine how this is achieved. With a Nightingale ward each side of the ward could be looked after by a team of nurses. A ward that has been upgraded and made into bays can be divided in the same way. Wards consisting of small rooms can be divided room by room.

The workload may be divided equally between the teams, especially if patients are admitted directly to empty beds which are not forever being moved. If for any reason the high-dependency patients are nursed in one part of the ward – for example, because of limited oxygen and suction points, or if part of the ward offers better observation of patients – then the team caring for the high-dependency patients will require additional nurses of varying experience.

Time is necessary in order that a relationship between patient and nurse can be established. Therefore it is beneficial to all if the same nurses look after the same patients. This is possible with team nursing, although it may be necessary from time to time to move patients from one part of the ward to another, depending on the facilities available in the ward. It is much easier to maintain some stability in the more modern wards consisting of four- or six-bedded rooms and single rooms. When nurses look after the same group of patients for a period of time problems may occur if a personality conflict develops or if the patient becomes too dependent on the same nurse. It may limit the nurse's experience and isolate her from the rest of the ward. Notwithstanding, the establishment of a secure nurse–patient relationship is the foundation of total patient care, and these difficulties can be overcome.

A team may consist of qualified nurses of different grades, student nurses, support workers and nursing auxiliaries. It is possible to plan the duty rota ensuring that the same team of nurses looks after the same patients at all times. This is achieved by covering the ward with the sister or charge nurse and senior staff nurses and then dividing the remainder of the staff into teams, with an even skill mix (see Table 6.2). This can be displayed as it is or transcribed onto a chart devised for the individual ward (see Table 6.3). Some sisters or charge nurses allocate the teams each day but this tends to give a lack of continuity and defeats the objective.

When planning duty rotas, internal rotation of staff to night duty can cause problems of continuity. These must be coordinated by the sister or charge nurse or by using a deputy team leader.

The team leader

The ward sister or charge nurse appoints the team leaders and must adequately prepare them for their roles. For example, on coming to the ward they may need a period of orientation to team nursing if this method of patient care is new to them. Each team leader is responsible to the ward sister or charge nurse.

The responsibilities the team leaders must assume are:

(1) To assign the team members to their patients. The support workers should be capable of caring for a small number of convalescent and ambulant patients under the guidance of the team leader. However, depending on the type of ward, the team leader may prefer to assign the support worker to assist one or two nurses in the team, but this will depend on staff available.

(2) To ensure that each nurse has a patient-orientated as opposed to a task-orientated approach, giving individualized care.

(3) To participate in patient care by having their own patients within the team.

Table 6.2 Duty Rota (day shifts).

Ward:				Week commencing:			
	Mon	Tues	Wed	Thurs	Fri	Sat	Sun
Sister	M	E	M	E	M	DO	DO
Staff nurse	DO	DO	E	M	E	M	E
Staff nurse	E	M	M Rm 1–4	DO	DO	E	M
Rooms 1–4							
Staff nurse	M	E	E	M	M	DO	DO
Staff nurse	M	DO	DO	E	E	M	E
3rd year student	E	M	E	M	M	DO	DO
3rd year student	E	M	M	DO	DO	E	M
Support worker	M	E	M	E	M	DO	DO
Support worker	DO	DO	E	M	DO	E	M
Nursing auxiliary	07.30– 13.30	07.30– 13.30	DO	DO	16.30– 21.30	07.30– 13.30	DO
Rooms 5–8							
Staff nurse	E	M	E	M	M	DO	DO
Staff nurse	Do	17.00– 21.30	07.30– 13.00	DO	DO	17.00– 21.30	07.30– 13.00
Enrolled nurse	M	DO	DO	E	E	M	E
3rd year student	DO	E	E	M	DO	E	M
Support worker	M	M	DO	DO	E	M	E
Support worker	DO	DO	07.30– 13.00	07.30– 13.00	07.30– 13.00	DO	16.30– 21.30 Rm 1–4
Nursing auxiliary	16.30– 21.30	16.30– 21.30	DO	16.30– 21.30	16.30– 21.30	DO	DO
Totals Morning	7	6	6	7	6	5	5
Evening	5	6	6	5	6	5	5

M—Morning   E—Evening Shift   DO—Day off

(4) To plan patient care together with the nurse concerned, after completing a round of the patients.

(5) To update the care plans with the nurse concerned and involving the patient.

(6) To ensure that nursing needs and medical requirements are met.

(7) To assess the effectiveness of care.

(8) To supervise and support the team members.

(9) To ensure that the student nurses in the team have the opportunity to learn, consolidate their skills and learn new skills.

Table 6.3 Plan for allocation of nurses (day shifts)

Ward:

				Week commencing:			
	Mon	Tues	Wed	Thurs	Fri	Sat	Sun
Morning/ Afternoon							
Rooms 1–4	Staff nurse Staff nurse Support worker	3rd year student 3rd year student Nursing auxiliary	Staff nurse 3rd year student Support worker	Staff nurse 3rd year student Support worker	Staff nurse 3rd year student Support worker	Staff nurse Nursing auxiliary	3rd year student Support worker
Rooms 5–8	Enrolled nurse Support worker Nursing auxiliary	Staff nurse Support worker	Staff nurse Support worker	Staff nurse 3rd year student	Staff nurse Support worker	Enrolled nurse Ssupport worker	Staff nurse 3rd year student
Afternoon/ Evening							
Rooms 1–4	3rd year student 3rd year student	Staff nurse Support worker	Staff nurse 3rd year student	Staff nurse Support worker	Staff nurse Nursing auxiliary	3rd yeat student Support worker	Staff nurse Support worker
Rooms 5–8	Staff nurse Nursing auxiliary	Staff nurse 3rd year student	Staff nurse 3rd year student	Enrolled nurse Nursing auxiliary	Enrolled nurse Nursing anxiliary	Staff nurse 3rd year student	Enrolled nurse Support worker

(10) To ensure that personality conflicts which may occasionally arise between patient and nurse are resolved speedily.

(11) To keep the ward sister or charge nurse informed of changes.

(12) To ensure that nursing records are maintained and completed accurately, including all the necessary information.

(13) To maintain a clean and safe environment.

(14) To ensure that the patients are kept well-informed about their care.

(15) To act as role model or mentor for more junior nurses.

Patient allocation, or assignment

Patient allocation is the allocation by the sister or charge nurse of one or sometimes two nurses to a group of patients, allowing the nurse to organize and carry out the care required by the patients for a span of duty. Again, the aim is to focus attention on the patients and the care they require to fulfil their needs and to overcome their nursing problems, as opposed to completion of tasks and fitting the patient into the ward routine.

Patient allocation may be achieved in a team nursing setting as previously described. In this case the team leader will assign the nurses to the patients. Alternatively, nurses on duty may be assigned to their patients by the ward sister or charge nurse who assesses the capability of each nurse. Support workers may be assigned their own patients as mentioned earlier or may be assigned to work with one or more nurses.

With this method of ward organization the nurses are responsible to the ward sister or charge nurse and assess their patients' needs, plan their care and then implement the care plan. They also evaluate the effectiveness of the care. The ward sister or charge nurse is available to assist in these activities and to provide support and supervision.

The groups of patients may be much smaller than those in team nursing. The method by which the ward is divided up will depend on the layout of the ward; wards with small rooms are much easier to cope with than are Nightingale wards. With this system it is more difficult to plan for each nurse to look after the same patients for any length of time because of days off, holidays and shifts, and the assignment of nurses to patients is easier on a daily basis. However, it can be planned ahead with careful thought and an allocation sheet used on similar lines to Table 6.3.

When student nurses are allocated to their own group of patients it must be made absolutely clear to them that they are responsible to the trained nurse with whom they are working and that they must discuss any changes of plan or any problems. On the other hand, if the sister or charge nurse had allocated them to their patients, he or she must be available and approachable to them and before assigning them to their patients must assess their capabilities and ensure that they know what is expected of them, what care is required by the patients and the boundaries of their responsibility.

The trained nurse allocated to a group of patients has much more autonomy and will deal with the patients' problems, for example, the nurse will liaise with the doctor if a patient's analgesia needs reviewing. This aspect makes it essential for the trained nurse to keep the ward sister or charge nurse fully informed, and time for effective communication should be worked into the daily plan.

Primary nursing

Primary nursing personalizes care on a one-to-one basis, from the time of admission to hospital until discharge.

Manthey (1973) states that primary nursing is a delivery system designed to allocate 24-hour responsibility for each patient's care to one individual. She goes on to say that high-quality nursing care should be the goal of every nurse – this means individualized care which is humane, competent, comprehensive and continuous. Primary nursing achieves this as it is a holistic model of care consisting of policies, procedures, relationships, behaviours, attitudes and competencies.

The ward sister or charge nurse assigns each patient to a named trained nurse, thereby giving trained nurses individual accountability for the nursing care of the patients assigned to them for the whole of their period of hospitalization. Some practitioners regard this as total responsibility for the patient both on- and off-duty, others do not. Therefore local policy should be quite clear.

The primary nurse becomes responsible for:

(1) Assessing the patient's nursing needs
(2) Planning the patient's care for each 24-hour period
(3) Setting goals with full involvement of the patient
(4) Providing the patient's care whilst on duty
(5) Evaluating the patient's care
(6) Teaching the patient and/or relatives
(7) Liaising with the doctor and other health care workers
(8) Planning discharge
(9) Communicating effectively both verbally and in writing so that care can continue as planned
(10) Acting as a secondary or associate nurse for other patients.

Identified secondary or associate nurses, who are other trained nurses, or student nurses, will continue the patient's care when the primary nurse is off-duty. This is on the lines of team nursing or patient allocation, but the primary nurse's plan of care is followed and she or he remains accountable.

If the ward is organized on the team nursing system, it is logical that one of the trained nurses in the team to which a particular patient is assigned becomes that patient's named primary nurse. Alternatively, if the ward nursing staff are divided into small teams, each team, responsible for a small group of patients, could consist of a primary nurse plus associate nurses with support workers and nursing auxiliaries.

If primary nursing is to be effective there must be certain criteria laid down and agreed. These might include, for example:

(1) A willingness of all trained nurses to accept full responsibility for a high standard of care.
(2) The level of trained nurses is such that, if possible each nurse has only five or six primary patients at a time but this may vary with the degree of dependency of the patients.
(3) A means of identifying immediately a patient's primary nurse, e.g. a chart (see Table 6.4).
(4) The primary nurse must be on duty when her or his allocated patient is admitted.

Table 6.4 Primary nursing – allocating patients to nurses.

Ward:	
Sister Merrill:	Mrs Palm
	Mrs Ash
	Mr Pine
Staff Nurse Pearce:	Mr Willow
	Miss Beech
	Mr Grove
	Mr Hawthorn
Staff Nurse Lynch:	Mrs Cherry
	Mr Larch
	Miss Woods
Staff Nurse Fenner:	Mr Lime
	Mr Elm
	Ms Rowan
	Mrs Forrest

(5) Support, leadership and continuing education must be provided by the sister or charge nurse.

(6) If a personality clash arises between patient and nurse the assignment must be discussed with both and changed if necessary.

(7) Supervision by the sister or charge nurse to ensure that written and verbal communication is of a very high standard, e.g. that care plans are written and up-to-date so that the nurse who takes over in the absence of the primary nurse knows about the patient and the care required.

With a primary nursing system the ward sister or charge nurse may also be allocated two or three patients, thus demonstrating that she or he is also a practitioner.

In achieving individualized care primary nursing goes further than team nursing or patient allocation, but is a system of ward organization that can be incorporated into both these organization systems.

The role of the nurse in charge

Team nursing and patient allocation

The organizational role of the sister or charge nurse will be similar for team nursing and patient allocation. They must ensure:

(1) Clear, logical guidelines for the pattern of the patients' day and the chosen method of organizing patient care are agreed by the team and made available.

(2) Awareness by the nursing staff of the patients for whom they are responsible, and the care required.

(3) Awareness by the nursing staff of what is expected of them and their limits of responsibility – that is, the extent of involvement in the care of the patient and in decision-making.

(4) Leadership, organization, supervision, and coordination of the ward nursing team.

(5) Delegation of care to the nurse concerned.

(6) Involvement of the nurse concerned in decision-making, even if that nurse is not able to make major decisions alone.

(7) Definition of areas of responsibility at times when there might be confusion, for example, during overlap of shifts.

(8) Continuation of care, day to night and night to day, valuing the contribution of night as well as day nurses, by liaising with the

night sister or charge nurse and showing positive encouragement
to the night nursing team.

(9)   A round of all patients at the beginning of the shift, either alone or
        with the nurse concerned, in order to assess patient needs.

(10)   Adequate and frequent opportunities are allowed for the ward
        nursing team to communicate with each other in order to avoid
        constant interruptions, and to enable them to pass on all relevant
        information so that everyone, especially the sister or charge nurse
        is kept fully informed. There must be frequent reports, the time
        involved not necessarily great, and it is essential that there is a
        brief report or handover at each change of staff.

        Ideally at each stage the nurse responsible for the patients is in
        the best position to give the report. However, this will need to be
        adapted according to the demands of the ward, although the nurse
        responsible for patient care must have at least one opportunity a
        day to report back to the ward sister or charge nurse, who must
        make sure that the report times are always adhered to, even when
        the ward is very busy.

(11)   Nurses are individually held accountable for the care they give.
        This is accomplished by ensuring that they have had an opportu-
        nity to report back to the sister or charge nurse as described
        above.

(12)   The sister or charge nurse encourages the nurses to keep
        themselves informed about all the patients in the ward so that,
        in an emergency, swift action can be taken by the nurse nearest at
        hand. Obviously, the nurse will have a much deeper knowledge of
        her or his own patients.

Primary nursing

If primary nursing is the chosen method of ward organization the ward
sister or charge nurse has more of an enabling and coordinating role. She
or he must:

(1)   Ensure that all staff understand the philosophy of primary nursing
        and accept it.

(2)   Coordinate the activities of the ward.

(3)   Plan duty rotas so that the associate nurse is able to deputize for
        the primary nurse.

(4)   Maintain the system.

(5)   Allocate patients to primary nurses together with delegation of
        decision-making.

(6)   Organize the allocation of patients to associate nurses.

(7) Ensure that each primary nurse is carrying a fair workload.

(8) Give supervision and support to primary nurses and less experienced primary nurses.

(9) Act as consultant and resource person to other members of the ward team.

(10) Instruct and educate those new to the ward.

(11) Maintain cohesiveness and communication within the nursing team.

(12) Monitor effectiveness of care.

(13) Agree and set standards of care for the ward with the nursing team.

(14) Act as a link between doctors, other health care workers and the primary nurse in the absence of the latter or if she or he is involved in care giving and is not able to be released.

(15) Provide continuity for the ward team by ensuring good communication, especially in the absence of the primary nurse.

(16) Validate care plans with the primary nurse to ensure they meet the patients' needs.

(17) Act as a role model.

(18) Act as a teacher and develop staff.

(19) Provide psychological support for staff and ensure all team members feel valued.

(20) If has own case-load, assess needs of patients on an on-going basis, spend time with them but may need to accept that most of their care will be given by associate nurses, with whom there will need to be very close liaison.

Continued involvement with the other patients on the ward is maintained.

A further benefit of primary nursing is that head-nurses are learning to make patient rounds which are centred more on knowing patients as persons and keeping abreast of changes in their conditions than on administrative checkups to see whether a nursing procedure has been completed or a piece of equipment repaired. These rounds, vitally important both to supplement factual information which the head-nurse has received for change of shift reports and to keep her abreast of staff–patient relationships, help her in assigning care and in the counselling of staff members. The head-nurse remains the pre-eminent unit leader.

(Manthey 1973)

Each sister or charge nurse will want to organize the nursing team to the best advantage of both patients and staff. This will mean taking into account the demand of the ward, the average staffing levels of the ward and the ratio of trained to untrained nurses. It may mean trying out different methods of ward organization before deciding on the best method for the ward.

Before implementing any change in the organization of the ward, whether it is the organization of the patients' day or the organization of the nursing team, there are two principles that must be followed.

First, the whole team must believe the principles of the new system are right for the ward and be prepared to work towards them. This means that the sister or charge nurse must have full discussion and reach agreement with all the staff involved before embarking on implementation; allow time not only to listen to staff's problems and answer their questions but to inform other people who are likely to be affected – clinical nurse manager, physiotherapist, doctors, social worker. Obviously, if the change is within team nursing, patient allocation or primary nursing, the preparation will be less involved than when changing from job allocation.

Second, the sister or charge nurse must provide strong leadership and be prepared to supervise and coordinate activities.

The optimum time to change is when the least number of staff are on holiday, or when the staffing levels are above average and there are more senior nurses in the team. When the pressures build up and situations become stressful the sister or charge nurse must encourage and support the nurses so that they are not tempted to revert to the former method of organization. Full discussion with the clinical nurse manager should ensure support and encouragement for the nursing team when the sister or charge nurse is off-duty.

Planning duty rotas

As stated earlier in this chapter, planning duty rotas can be a difficult job – especially when continuity of patient care is to be considered, and internal rotation to night duty is practised. However, there are some hints and tips which, from the authors' experience, might help.

The aim of a well-planned duty rota is to ensure that the ward is adequately staffed at all times with a trained nurse in charge of each shift and a balance of grades of staff. It must be planned so that the staff are in the right place at the right time. It must, however, be structured in such a way that it not only covers the ward effectively but is also fair to the staff. It is essential to plan well ahead so that team members can plan for their off-duty time. If planned in advance it will give the clinical nurse manager an indication of when help is required from the relief pool or nurses bank.

When planning the rota consideration must be given to:

- RGN-cover for the ward for each shift
- Balance of senior and junior staff
- Balance of trained and untrained staff
- Continuity from one day to the next, especially for the most senior staff, following days-off and holidays
- Busier days – theatre days, emergency take days
- Proper cover of evenings and weekends as well as the morning shift
- Sharing weekends off, and considering the financial implications when planning the rota for weekends and public holidays, relating the possible workload to the level of staff required to achieve a safe level of care
- Preference for days-off together or split days-off
- Special requests
- Set days for some part-time staff
- Night cover if internal rotation to night duty is practised.

A skeleton plan is made in pencil to allow alterations, and the steps that may be taken when building up the plan are:

(1) List names in order of seniority.
(2) Put special requests in ink to avoid erasure (see Table 6.6).
(3) Insert days off, noting busier days. It is important not to have too many nurses off-duty at the same time. An aid in obtaining an even distribution of staff throughout the week is to total the number of days-off required in one week and divide by seven. This gives the approximate number of nurses who can be off-duty on any one day (see Table 6.5).

    When writing in days-off, refer to the previous rota so that days-off are reasonably spaced and weekends off are shared (see Table 6.5).
(4) Add, in ink, those nurses who work set shifts. This will usually be some or all of the part-time staff (see Table 6.6).
(5) Add the shifts, balancing senior and junior nurses on each shift, ensuring that there is a senior nurse on duty to take charge, and that the trained nurses are evenly balanced (see Table 6.7).

    Most people prefer an early duty before, and a late duty after days-off. If a senior nurse requests to work a morning shift after days-off or if this is more suitable to the ward, it is preferable if that nurse is not in charge of the ward that particular morning, so that

Table 6.5 Duty rota showing 37 days-off to be allocated in one week

Ward:				Week commencing:			
	Mon	Tues	Wed	Thurs	Fri	Sat	Sun
Sister						DO	DO
Staff nurse	DO	DO					
Staff nurse	←			NIGHT DUTY			→
Staff nurse				DO	DO		
Staff nurse	←			NIGHTS OFF			→
Staff nurse	←			NIGHT DUTY			→
Staff nurse		DO	DO				
Staff nurse						DO	DO
Staff nurse	←			NIGHTS OFF			→
Staff nurse				DO	DO		
Staff nurse			DO	DO			
Enrolled nurse		DO	DO				
Enrolled nurse						DO	DO
3rd year student				DO	DO		
3rd year student	DO				DO		
3rd year student						DO	DO
Support worker	DO	DO			DO		
Support worker	←			NIGHT DUTY			→
Support worker	DO	DO	DO	DO			
Support worker		DO	DO				
Support worker	←			ANNUAL LEAVE			→
Support worker	DO						DO
Nursing auxiliary	←			NIGHTS OFF			→
Nursing auxiliary						DO	DO
Total Days off Each Day	5	6	5	5	5	5	6

DO – Day off

better continuity of care is achieved. However, if the returning nurse is the only trained nurse on duty then she or he will have to fulfil this role, as long as there is another nurse on duty able to bring her or him up-to-date.

(6) Total the number of staff on duty for each shift (see Table 6.7).

It may be found that it is easier to plan the rota on a fortnightly or monthly basis. In some hospitals the rota may be a fixed one with new staff being allocated to a line of off-duty.

If team nursing is practised the teams can be arranged when the rota is planned, after the senior staff's duties have been arranged, so that the ward is covered by a senior trained nurse.

Table 6.6 Duty rota with special requests and set shifts added

Ward:				Week commencing:			
	Mon	Tues	Wed	Thurs	Fri	Sat	Sun
Sister						DO	DO
Staff nurse	DO	DO					
Staff nurse	←			NIGHT DUTY			→
Staff nurse				DO	DO		
Staff nurse	←			NIGHTS OFF			→
Staff nurse	←			NIGHT DUTY			→
Staff nurse		DO	DO				
Staff nurse		M^R	E^R			DO	DO
Staff nurse	←			NIGHTS OFF			→
Staff nurse				DO	DO		
Staff nurse		DO	DO				
Enrolled nurse	07.30–13.30	DO	DO	16.00–21.30	16.00–21.30	07.30–13.30	16.00–21.30
Enrolled nurse						DO	DO
3rd year student			M^R	DO	DO		
3rd year student	DO				DO^R	E^R	
3rd year student					M^R	DO^R	DO^R
Support worker	DO	DO	07.30–13.30	07.30–13.30	DO	07.30–13.30	07.30–13.30
Support worker	←			NIGHT DUTY			→
Support worker	DO	DO	DO	DO	16.00–21.30	16.00–21.30	16.00–21.30
Support worker		DO	DO				
Support worker	←			ANNUAL LEAVE			→
Support worker	DO						DO
Nursing auxiliary	←			NIGHTS OFF			→
Nursing auxiliary						DO	DO
	5	6	5	5	5	5	6

R – Request   M – Morning Shift   E – Evening Shift   DO – Day Off

If it is the practice to cover the night shift by internal rotation this is best achieved by putting in nights to be covered and nights-off at the same time as planning the days-off. The total number of nights covered and nights-off are added to the total number of days-off required in order to ascertain the number of nurses able to be away each day.

If deemed necessary to alter the rota those affected must be notified. If it becomes difficult to cover the ward adequately, a nurse who normally works set hours might be willing to change days-off or a shift if approached beforehand.

Table 6.7 Duty rota completed

Ward:				Week commencing:			
	Mon	Tues	Wed	Thurs	Fri	Sat	Sun
Sister	M	E	M	E	M	DO	DO
Staff nurse	DO	DO	E	M	E	M	E
Staff nurse	◄——————— NIGHT DUTY ———————►						
Staff nurse	E	M	M	DO	DO	E	M
Staff nurse	◄——————— NIGHTS OFF ———————►						
Staff nurse	◄——————— NIGHT DUTY ———————►						
Staff nurse	M	DO	DO	E	E	M	E
Staff nurse	E	M^R	E^R	M	M	DO	DO
Staff nurse	◄——————— NIGHTS OFF ———————►						
Staff nurse	M	E	M	DO	DO	E	M
Staff nurse	E	M	DO	DO	E	M	E
Enrolled nurse	07.30–13.30	DO	DO	16.00–21.30	16.00–21.30	07.30–13.30	16.00–21.30
Enrolled nurse	E	M	E	M	M	DO	DO
3rd year student	M	E	M^R	DO	DO	E	M
3rd year student	DO	E	E	M	DO^R	E^R	M
3rd year student	E	M	M	E	M^R	DO^R	DO^R
Support worker	DO	DO	07.30–13.30	07.30–13.30	DO	07.30–13.30	07.30–13.30
Support worker	◄——————— NIGHT DUTY ———————►						
Support worker	DO	DO	DO	DO	16.00–21.30	16.00–21.30	16.00–21.30
Support worker	M	DO	DO	E	M	M	E
Support worker	◄——————— ANNUAL LEAVE ———————►						
Support worker	DO	E	M	M	M	M	DO
Nursing auxiliary	◄——————— NIGHTS OFF ———————►						
Nursing auxiliary	M	M	E	M	M	DO	DO
	5	6	5	5	5	5	6
TOTALS – Morning:	7	6	7	7	7	7	6
Evening:	5	5	5	5	5	5	5
Night:	3	3	3	3	3	3	3

R – Request   M – Morning Shift   E – Evening Shift   DO – Day Off

So long as the trained staff levels permit, senior part-time trained nurses may be used as a back-up and support the more junior trained nurses, and not left in charge of the ward except in an emergency situation. The part-time staff nurse may not have the continuity of patient care to enable her or him to take charge effectively, although they can be used as team leaders.

Holidays

The sister or charge nurse should be aware of the holiday entitlement of each of the permanent nurses, who should also be fully aware of the holidays allocated to them. Holiday entitlements are listed in the Whitley Council Handbook, with a set entitlement for full-time staff.

It should be noted that salaries and conditions of service for staff can be set by hospital Trusts rather than following Whitley Council agreements.

Annual leave entitlements

- Full-time trained nurses   5 weeks plus public holidays
- Part-time trained nurses   6½ weeks plus an extra day for each public holiday introduced since 1978 (option A) or 5 weeks plus a day in lieu for each public holiday which is worked (option B).
- Full-time nursing auxiliaries   4 weeks plus public holidays
- Part-time nursing auxiliaries   5½ weeks plus an extra day for each public holiday introduced since 1978 (option A) or 4 weeks plus a day in lieu for each public holiday which is worked (option B). Nursing auxiliaries are also entitled to long service days off after completing 5, then 10 years service. These are given in proportion to hours worked and are confirmed by the personnel department. If there is any doubt about either annual leave or long service leave it should be discussed with the clinical nurse manager.
- All part-time staff have a choice of either option A or B on commencing employment which cannot be renegotiated unless there is a change in contract.

Nurses should be encouraged to plan ahead for their holidays. Only a certain number of staff should be allowed to take their holidays at the same time. The number is usually agreed between the sister or charge nurse and the clinical nurse manager, after considering the peaks and troughs in the workload throughout the coming year.

Manpower is the largest resource within the ward and it is vital, therefore, to use it efficiently, e.g. when planning staff holidays, the peaks and troughs in the ward workload should, if possible, be taken into account. Shift times are usually specified by the hospital's nursing management but individual units should aim to minimise staff overlap if possible. When planning duty rotas, the number of staff for each shift must be critically appraised, and based on the forecasted needs of the patients, especially at weekends and public holidays, because of the cost implication. Financial consideration should never, be at the expense of patient care, a balance between the two being maintained at all times.

Control of environment

Florence Nightingale said that hospitals should do the sick no harm. This can be extended to include visitors and also staff. Part of the ward sister's or charge nurse's responsibility is to control the environment of the ward so that patients are as comfortable as possible and that patients, visitors and staff are safe. The most important environment factors to be considered are:

- Safety
- Ventilation
- Light
- Cleanliness
- Control of noise
- Privacy

Although some of these are not solely the responsibility of the sister or charge nurse, if there is a fault – for example, a problem with central heating – the problem must be brought to the attention of the department concerned, by the appropriate requisition. If urgent attention is indicated it is usually acceptable to telephone the department concerned and follow this with a requisition. Persistent difficulties should be discussed with the head of the appropriate department or clinical nurse manager.

Summary

The day-to-day organization of the ward comprises a multitude of activities ranging from the organization of the patients' day to developing effective methods of organizing the way in which the nurses work and in which patients each receive the most appropriate care. It includes planning off-duty rotas and holidays, and ensuring that patients have a safe and hospitable hospital environment. This chapter has aimed to provide some hints and guidance for achieving these tasks. It has not used many direct references, and much of the material comes from the authors' own experiences as well as from a variety of literary sources. For this reason, the references and recommended reading list have been combined at the end of the chapter.

Topics for discussion

1. Models for nursing care:
Choose a patient currently in your care, and, using a model other than

the one you currently use, attempt to draw up a care plan for one or two identified patient problems. How does this care plan differ from the one in use on your ward? Would the difference have any impact on the patient or his response to his care?

2. Imagine you are a patient admitted to hospital with a fractured femur following a car accident. The ward into which you are admitted uses task allocation as the method of organizing the nursing team. Discuss the advantages and disadvantages you would find with this system, assuming your hospital stay lasts about 10 days. Contrast these with the advantages and disadvantages you might find if patient allocation or primary nursing was in operation.

3. Using Table 6.7, work out ways in which you could adequately cover the ward if one of the senior staff nurses on day duty goes off sick with a bad back and is unlikely to return to work for two weeks.

4. The nursing management of the hospital want to change the nurses' shift patterns in order to reduce the two-hour staff overlap in the afternoon to $^{3}/_{4}$ hour. You have been asked for suggestions for how this might be achieved. What would your response be, and how would you implement the change in order to minimize the staff disruption, both emotional and practical?

References and Recommended Reading

Brown, R.A. (1989) *Individualised Care: The role of the Ward Sister*, RCN Research series, Scutari Press, Harrow

Cartwright, A. (1964) *Human Relations and Hospital Care*. Routledge and Kegan Paul, London.

Cavanagh, S. (1991) *Orem's Model in Action* MacMillan, London.

Chapman, C.M. (1985) *Theory of Nursing: Practical Application*. Harper and Row, London.

Chavasse, J. (1981) From task assignment to patient allocation – A change evaluation *Journal of Advanced Nursing*, 6, 137–45.

Ersser, S. & Tutton, E. (ed.) (1991) *Primary Nursing in Perspective*. Scutari, London.

Hegyvary, S.T. (1982) *The Change to Primary Nursing*. Mosby, St. Louis, Missouri.

Henderson, V. (1966) *The Nature of Nursing: A Definition and its Implication, Practice, Research and Education*. Macmillan, New York.

Henderson, V. (1968) *Basic Principles of Nursing Care*. International Council of Nurses, Basel. Karger, London and Geneva.

Hunt, J.M. & Marks-Maran, D.J. (1986) Nursing care plans in *The Nursing Process At Work*. (2nd ed) Education for Care Series, H.M. and M. Publishers.

Kershaw, B. & Salvage, J. (ed) *Models for Nursing*. Wiley, Chichester.

Kratz, C. (ed) (1979) *The Nursing Process – a Scientific Approach to Nursing Care*. C.V. Mosby Co, London.

Kron, T. (1987) *The Management of Patient Care: Putting Leadership Skills to Work* (6th ed). W.B. Saunders Co, Philadelphia.

McFarlane, J.K. (1976) A charter for caring (The Royal College of Nursing Lecture 1975). *Journal of Advanced Nursing* **1**, 187–96.

McFarlane Baroness of Llandaff, & Castledine, G. (1982) *The Practice of Nursing Using The Nursing Process*. C.V. Mosby Co., London.

Manthey, M. (1973) Primary Nursing is Alive and Well in the Hospital. *American Journal of Nursing* **73**, 1, 83–7.

Manthey, M. (1980) *The Practice of Primary Nursing* Blackwell Scientific Publications Inc, Boston.

Maslow, A.H. (1962) *Towards a Psychology of Being*. Van Nostrand, New Jersey.

Matthews, A. (1975) Patient Allocation – a Review. *Nursing Times Occasional Papers*, July pp. 65–69.

Metcalfe, C.A. (1982) *A study of a change in the method of organizing the delivery of nursing care in a ward of a maternity hospital*. Unpublished PhD Thesis, University of Manchester.

Newton, C. (1991) *The Roper–Logan–Tierney Model in Action* Macmillan, London.

Nightingale, F. (1974 – original 1859) *Notes on Nursing*. Blackie, London.

Orem, D. (1985) *Nursing: Concepts of Practice*. McGraw Hill, New York.

Pearson, A. (ed.) (1988) *Primary Nursing*. Nursing in the Burford and Oxford Nursing Development Units. Croom Helm, London.

Pearson, A. & Vaughan, B. (1986) *Nursing Models for Practice*. Heinemann, London.

Pembrey, S. (1975) From work routines to patient assignment. *Nursing Times* **72** (45) Nov. 6. pp. 1768–72.

Report of a Seminar for Fellows of the Royal College of Nursing (1980) *Accountability in Nursing*.

Riehl, J.P. & Roy, C. (eds) (1980) *Conceptual Models for Nursing Practice*. Appleton–Century–Crofts, New York.

Roper, N. (1982) *Principles of Nursing*. Churchill Livingstone, Edinburgh.

Tierney, A.J. (ed.) (1986) Clinical nursing practice. *Recent Advances in Nursing*. **14**. Churchill Livingstone, Edinburgh.

Webb, C. (1981) Classification and framing: a sociological analysis of task-centred nursing and the nursing process *Journal of Advanced Nursing*, **6**, 369–76.

Wright, S.G. (ed.) (1990) *My Patient, My Nurse: a guide to primary nursing*. Scutari, London.

Chapter 7
Preparation for inpatient care

Admission to hospital, as an outpatient or an inpatient, can be a traumatic experience for patients and their relatives. People react in different ways but when in hospital most patients want the nurses to care for them and to treat and respect them as human beings at a very stressful and uncertain time of their lives. The way in which the patients adapt to this new situation is partly dependent on the way the nursing team receives them into the department or the ward.

First impressions are usually lasting impressions. The reception the patient receives from the nursing staff on arrival in the outpatient department or in the ward usually has a lasting effect.

Effect of and reaction to hospitalization

The hospital setting is strange and frightening. Most people, when sick, are nursed in their own homes, and it is natural to be afraid of strangers, new surroundings and new situations. These encounters can lead to anxiety and stress. Illness can threaten our very existence. Previous experience of being a hospital patient may reduce or increase anxiety on subsequent admissions.

Anxiety and stress

Patients who feel very ill on admission to hospital are less likely to feel anxious. They tend to feel a sense of relief. The patients who are not feeling ill, however, usually experience much anxiety (Wilson Barnett, 1979).

Causes of anxiety

Most people are terrified at the thought of going to hospital and arrive in a hypersensitive state. On admission to hospital anxiety can be caused

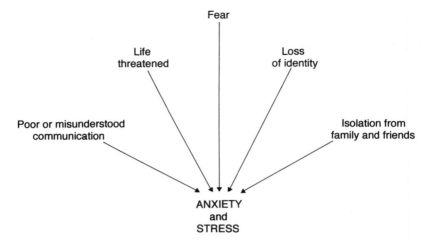

Fig. 7.1   Causes of stress and anxiety.

by many things. (Fig. 7.1.) Fear of the unknown will create anxiety in most people. This may include fear of:

- Loss of independence
- Loss of dignity
- Lack of information
- Information not understood or only part understood
- Hospital environment
- Being away from the family
- Seeing very ill patients
- Lack of knowledge of the staff in various uniforms
- Lack of knowledge of the routine
- Loss of employment
- Strange apparatus
- Anaesthesia, which may be related to previous experience of mask and ether
- Tests, painful procedures, surgery
- Injections
- Pain and death

Other factors which contribute towards anxiety are:

- Loss of identity
- Loss of control of one's destiny
- Disruption of routine
- Lack of knowledge of available facilities

- Lack of knowledge of oneself as a patient
- Being away from work
- Reduction in income
- Missing friends
- Boredom
- Worry about spouse/partner/family
- Failure to be involved in one's care
- Failure to be involved in decisions affecting oneself
- Past experience of hospitals.

One of the most common complaints highlighted in many surveys, such as that of Cartwright (1964), is the patient's difficulty in obtaining information. This causes anxiety which, in turn, impairs communication. Stress will occur if patients receive inadequate information from doctors and nurses about tests, procedures, investigations, treatments and surgery. The use of strange medical terms and explanations or information which is ambiguous or evasive, will increase a patient's anxiety.

A patient who has had an unhappy experience in hospital, or one who suffers from agoraphobia or claustrophobia will obviously demonstrate a high level of anxiety.

Manifestations of anxiety

Fear and anxiety manifest themselves in different ways. An individual's reaction to illness and hospital will vary greatly but will be affected by the meaning of the illness to the patient and to his or her family, and its possible effects on future lifestyle. It is imperative that nurses know what reactions may occur and that they are aware of the patients' feelings and fears. If these reactions are recognized by the nursing team, their response to the patients can be adjusted to meet their individual needs so that recovery is enhanced.

Individuals experience anxiety when unsure about things, as in the case of a patient who is uncertain about what is going to take place at the time of operation, or is not able to control events. This can be experienced prior to anaesthesia. This leads to a feeling of helplessness and forms a major component of stress (Boore, 1978).

If adequate information is given to a patient preoperatively, stress is relieved which, in turn, reduces the level of postoperative pain. An example of this is telling the patient what is planned at the operation, explaining that there will be discomfort after the operation but this will be relieved by appropriate means (Hayward, 1975).

Many patients show their anxiety by being restless, tearful and unable to sleep. They may be too anxious to take in explanations. Some regress, becoming childlike and dependent on the staff. This often results in patients being very demanding. Other patients may become irrational, finicky, complaining, irritable or aggressive. Adult patients who are always complaining about the food, the treatment or the staff, may be desperately trying to cover up their anxiety and fear. Excessive joking and laughter may be an attempt to cover up fear. The laughter is often inappropriate. Some patients try to become the centre of attention. This is possibly because they are afraid to be left alone. On the other hand, elderly patients who live alone and feel unneeded may become quite demanding and dependent upon the nursing staff, trying to get the attention they feel they lacked at home. They may also appear more ill when their family visits, demonstrating the need for attention. They may even become incontinent of urine, and possibly faeces, to bring attention to themselves.

Most patients show gratitude and are thankful that something is being done for them. Others appear to be coping well, stating that everything is alright and that they have no worries. This may indicate a denial of reality. Others release their pent-up emotions and desires by being noisy or overly talkative, or even shouting. They may question treatment, and find it difficult to settle into the ward. If patients appear uncooperative it may be a sign that they are unable to verbalize their fears and problems, either because of their anxiety or because they are not articulate.

A feeling of depression may occur following admission to hospital. This may be more severe if the patient is already anxious because of the factors mentioned earlier. Those patients who have been, or who are likely to be in hospital for any length of time, are likely to become more depressed than those admitted for a relatively short stay. The patient who is not sure of the proposed length of stay, or who is ill-informed about proposed investigations and treatment, may show signs of depression.

Patients who are frequently admitted to hospital, those who are subjected to repeated investigations, surgical procedures, or treatments such as blood transfusions, and those who undergo prolonged treatments such as radiotherapy and chemotherapy are likely to have an increased level of anxiety and are more likely to show signs of depression. There is a tendency for some of these patients to be excessively demanding and appear 'hospitalized'.

Patients with life threatening or long term illness, especially if the breadwinner, may have a sense of guilt because they feel that they have let their partner and family down in some way.

Patients can become very bored, especially those who are subjected to enforced inactivity, for example, those on traction, or paralysed patients, and those whose treatment takes up a very small part of the day, but is spread out over many days, such as those having radio-therapy. Bored patients have more time to think about themselves and their illness and their level of anxiety may increase because of this.

Patients who are given conflicting information by nurses or doctors, such as time of operation or date of discharge, will become more anxious and possibly hostile.

Helping the patient adjust

The ward sister or charge nurse is the ideal person to assist the nursing team in helping the patient through this difficult time. From experience, she or he is able to recognize emotional disturbances caused by stress and anxiety and so can react with understanding. She or he has the important task of handing on these skills and guiding the nurse. The nursing team will take their lead from the sister, or charge nurse, therefore her or his approach to the situation must be one of kindness and understanding. If she or he is abrupt or hostile, and chastises the patients the nurses will do the same. If the sister or charge nurse remarks that Mr X is 'difficult' or a 'trouble maker' because he asks questions, is aggressive or complains, the nurses will do likewise and also tend to avoid the patient.

The sister or charge nurse should not be influenced by past experi-ences or their own ideals, in their attitude to the patients. For example, when the sister or charge nurse is a teetotaller she or he must not condemn the alcoholic patient, or when short of beds for emergency patients she or he must not criticize the patient admitted with a self-inflicted illness. The sister or charge nurse can help the staff by:

(1) Making them aware of the different reactions which can occur so that they can spot the warning signs.
(2) Making them aware of ways of reducing anxiety on admission to hospital, so that the patient is helped from admission.
(3) Being able to take a more conceptual view of a problem and so defuse potentially difficult situations.

Making staff aware of different reactions

If all nurses are aware of the ways in which a patient may react to admission to hospital they will be able to respond to the patient with understanding and empathy, rather than with criticism, especially if the patient is experiencing difficulty in adjusting. Informal talks and discus-sions with the ward sister or charge nurse will help the nurses to gain a better understanding of the effects of hospitalization.

Nurses tend to forget that hospitals are frightening places as they spend so much of their time in the hospital ward, therefore the nurse in charge should continue to remind them that most patients feel very nervous, and that many are terrified.

Aggressive people are often frightened and insecure (they attack before they can be attacked). The sister or charge nurse can help the nurses by explaining this to them. If a patient is showing aggressive tendencies it is essential to discover why. If patients are aware of the seriousness of their illness they may well react against society by adopting abnormal behaviour.

When a patient is aggressive, rude or demanding it is of help to the nursing team if the sister or charge nurse discusses with them the possible causes of patients' adverse responses. If they are made aware of some of the reasons for this response they may be able to come to terms with the patients' behaviour and help them through their illnesses. It also avoids patients being labelled 'difficult' or 'uncooperative'.

Mr Jacaranda, a 43-year-old Asian Ugandan, was receiving treatment for chronic myeloid leukaemia which then became acute myeloblastic leukaemia. He had been attending the outpatient department regularly and then required admission to the ward. When arranging his admission the doctor told a nurse that Mr Jacaranda tended to be rather difficult. Following admission, he settled very slowly, was demanding and miserable and appeared to require a high level of strong analgesia. Soon after his admission, the sister and the nursing team discussed Mr Jacaranda's position and the following facts became known:

1 Mr Jacaranda and his family had been turned out of Uganda and were trying to settle into a new country and a new home. His wife spoke very little English. His two eldest sons were taking important examinations at school.

2 He was a teacher and was trying to adjust to a new post, teaching 15-year-old boys.

3 He knew he had chronic myeloid leukaemia and realized that he was not making the progress he had expected.

It became obvious that Mr Jacaranda was frightened for himself and his family and he therefore reacted as he did. The discussion helped to change the attitude of the nursing team to him. They became much more understanding and accepted him for himself. He and his family were given help and support during repeated readmissions to the ward until the time that he died, with his family with him.

Ways of reducing anxiety on admission

The nursing team must be motivated and made aware of the patients' needs. Patients' anxiety on admission can be reduced (Fig. 7.2) by:

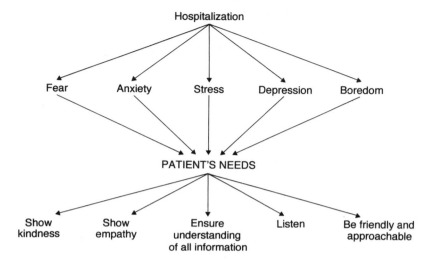

Fig. 7.2 Reaction to hospital and ways of helping the patient.

(1) Greeting patients with a smile and gentle voice and welcoming them by name.
(2) Introducing oneself by name and being friendly and approachable.
(3) Introducing patients to the nurse or nurses who will be responsible for their care.
(4) Introducing the patient to the other patients by name.
(5) Explaining the facilities on the ward – location of dayroom, toilet, bathroom, the patient–nurse call system, meal times, newspaper delivery times.
(6) Explaining what is expected of the patients – if and where they can smoke, if they can keep their day clothes and wear them, if they are to get into bed, if they may go out into the grounds or to the hospital shop.
(7) Explaining the ward routine.
(8) Giving information about visiting arrangements.
(9) Explaining the different uniforms and grades of staff. In many hospitals much of this information will be contained in the patients information booklet which is usually sent to the patient prior to admission. However, the information will need to be reinforced in many instances. Patients admitted as emergencies will not have had the opportunity to read the booklet, so will need to be given special consideration.
(10) Giving the patients explanations that they are able to understand about special equipment, tests, drugs, procedures, X-rays, treat-

ment, and never referring to anything as being 'only routine'. *Nothing is routine for the patient.*

All information must be related to the needs and expectations of the individual patient. It is imperative that the nurse is able to assess what the patient really wants to know (Abdellah & Levine, 1957).

(11) Warning the patients about possible side-effects of treatment but reassuring them that these can be minimized or controlled, for example, postoperative pain, effects of irradiation, effects of chemotherapy. It is extremely important that the correct information is given, and that all information given is fully understood.

(12) Involving the patients in any decision-making related to their care.

(13) Allowing the patients to wear day clothes and retain some of their personal possessions (wardrobes are not essential, as long as the patient has a bedside locker).

Mrs Palm, a spritely, 72-year-old housewife, was admitted to a Care of the Elderly assessment unit for investigation of increasing dyspnoea. On admission, all her clothes, including dressing gown, night dress and slippers, jewellery and money, were sent home. She was later transferred to another hospital, wearing clothes that belonged to the Care of the Elderly unit. She was most distressed and said that she felt as if her whole identity had been taken away when her clothing and personal possessions were taken from her. She began to wear her own clothes again and became happier and more relaxed.

(14) Giving the patients the opportunity to express their needs and fears, by carefully phrasing questions.

(15) Minimizing any embarrassment to the patient and preserving the patient's dignity.

Patients with urine drainage bags or Redivac drainage bottles may find these embarrassing, in which case they should be hidden from sight.

After admission, if patients still appear anxious they may find it helpful to talk about their illness and how it is affecting them. This is something that patients may find easier to talk over with nurses rather than other members of the health care team or their family.

Mr Gorse, a 65-year-old retired engineer, had made detailed plans with his wife to travel extensively following his retirement. However, two months after he had retired from a very demanding job he developed a chronic and debilitating illness. He realized that he would never be able to travel very far from home. This made him feel very angry and resentful and whilst in hospital he was demanding and uncooperative, and rude to his wife when she visited. He talked about his job, his plans and his bitter disappointment to the ward sister, who then relayed this to the nursing team. Mr Gorse was no longer rude, although he did become frustrated with himself, but the nursing team were able to give him the support and understanding he needed as they were aware of the effect of his illness on him.

Adjustment to hospital has been shown (Boore, J. 1978) to be mainly associated with making friends and becoming familiar with the people and procedures of the ward. The nurse who is aware of the patient's normal lifestyle is better able to assess problems and needs, and to foresee potential problems. This will also help the patient to adjust.

Communicating with patients' relatives and involving them

Sickness affects the family unit because it is an abnormal situation. It therefore causes great emotional trauma with which some people are better able to cope than others. Sometimes the family finds it difficult to function properly when one of its members is ill. Relatives may not act as they normally do. They find it difficult to assimilate what is said to them until they are able to come to terms with the consequences of the illness. As a guide, nurses should try to put themselves in the position of the relatives, and treat them as they would wish to be treated themselves. They will obviously follow the example of the ward sister or charge nurse.

The patient's relatives may react in a variety of ways when accompanying the patient to hospital or when visiting. They may show a sense of relief that treatment is being given. On the other hand, they may become hypersensitive and extremely anxious and frightened, worrying about the possible outcome of the illness.

Some sick people do ask their relatives not to send them to hospital but this becomes necessary when hospital treatment is indicated, or the family are no longer able to cope at home. Some relatives feel that they could have done more. In these situations they feel guilty and this sometimes shows itself as anger towards the hospital, doctors or nurses, or as a demanding, questioning approach. Relatives may also appear to be over-critical.

The same signs may be exhibited by relatives who are worried about the outcome of the illness, or those for whom hospitalization has other implications, such as financial or social. A woman with small children may be worried about coping with the children, or finding adequate money for food and bus fares, if her husband is in hospital for a long period.

Not all relatives react in the same way and most are helpful and understanding. Some people, however, do not show their distress and anxiety. This must not be mistaken for indifference and complacency. The way in which the individual reacts will depend on their personality, how they see the situation overall, and the problems hospitalization may create. The effects of hospitalization on relatives are very similar to those experienced by the patient which were discussed earlier in this chapter.

If given the opportunity, relatives can provide a lot of valuable information for the nursing team. Such information may include what the patient was like before becoming ill, any special likes or dislikes regarding food and drink, who usually helps at home, and any local authority services received. This sort of information will help the nurses to meet many of the patient's individual needs and plan for discharge home when the time comes.

The confidence of relatives must be gained. Explaining about visiting arrangements, special apparatus, things to bring, and so forth, gives the nurse an opportunity to talk with the relatives, who should then begin to feel more at ease. They will feel that the nurse understands them and wants to help. Often relatives need to talk to someone. Acting as counsellor to relatives is an important part of the nurse's role. It is important that relatives and friends understand that trained nurses, especially the sister or charge nurse, can be approached at any time.

When relatives are difficult and aggressive, the nurse should meet them with politeness and tact, never with aggression. Many seemingly aggressive relatives feel relieved to 'get things off their chests' if they find a sympathetic and understanding nurse. It is understandable if the widowed mother of a dying son is distraught and hostile and in need of support, or if the husband of a terminally ill mother of young children is antagonistic to the nursing staff whenever he visits. In these situations it is important that the ward sister or charge nurse makes sure that the nursing team understands the behaviours exhibited by relatives.

A high level of anxiety leads to defective communication, so it is essential that when talking to relatives everything is explained in a way they are able to understand. Relatives must be spoken to with respect for their level of intelligence and knowledge. It is essential to try to find out what they already know, but if in any doubt it is always better to assume that they have no knowledge of the subject and explain in detail.

Many terms used in hospital are not understood by the layman. Many people, for example, will not understand what myocardial infarction means, although they may know what a heart attack is. It is often necessary to repeat what has been said to relatives several times, perhaps in different ways, before they fully understand the situation. It must be remembered that when people are anxious and distraught it is very difficult for them to assimilate everything at once.

Correct information must always be given. If relatives receive conflicting information from the ward sister or charge nurse, the staff nurse or the doctor, they may become hostile. The ward sister or charge nurse has a responsibility to ensure that the relatives are fully informed and aware of the patient's general progress, or deterioration, possible transfer or discharge date, etc., but it is the responsibility of the doctor to explain in depth the medical details and treatment. The sister or charge nurse may need to make an appointment for the relatives to see the doctor. If it is felt that the relatives need to see a doctor straightaway it is the responsibility of the ward sister or charge nurse to ensure a meeting is arranged as soon as practicable, even if it is with the doctor on call. The ward sister is not there to protect the doctor from the relatives – all relatives have a right to see the doctor. When the doctor talks to relatives it is beneficial if a nurse is present so that the nursing team can be made aware of what has been said. This information is vital if clarification is needed at a later stage.

If a patient over the age of 16 years requests that relatives are not given any information this request must be respected. If the request seems unreasonable, however, it should be discussed carefully with the patient to see if this is really the patient's wish. It may be felt necessary to seek advice from the unit manager.

Patients and their relatives will need to talk with each other and share their thoughts and anxieties, and express their feelings for each other, and may appreciate privacy from time to time.

If a patient is distressed when the family visits, drawing the screens around the bed, or sometimes offering the privacy of the ward office if this is convenient, may be very beneficial. When it is necessary to nurse patients with bedrails in position for the sake of the patient's safety, it is far less distressing for relatives and friends if the bedrails are removed during the visiting period as long as a nurse is told when the visitors are leaving. This will enable patient and relatives to have more contact and to communicate better.

It can only do good if mothers, fathers, wives, husbands, or children are encouraged to assist with nursing care where indicated, and when it has been ascertained that this is the wish of both the patient and the relative. There are many instances when both patients and relatives will find strength and support if they are encouraged to participate. This may include assisting in the care of a child, learning how to assist a patient who is being rehabilitated prior to discharge, taking part in activities such as getting in and out of bed or a wheelchair, getting dressed, or fitting an artificial limb, and assisting in the care of the elderly or a terminally ill patient. Feeding helpless or disabled patients at mealtimes is another way of helping.

It is the nurse who usually takes the initiative and suggests that a relative might like to help, as most relatives tend to feel that once a patient is admitted to hospital the ward staff take over the care. However, if the ward nurses are aware that the ward sister or charge nurse favours relative participation and supports this, they will suggest to the relatives, where indicated, that they may like to assist in the patient's care, which, in many instances, they have been doing at home often for a long time prior to admission.

Children as patients

Any child who has the misfortune to go to hospital should not find the experience frightening if the time in hospital is made as happy as possible.

Children are often frightened by anything which is unfamiliar to them – people, uniforms, equipment – and must be helped by the nursing team to overcome these fears.

Nearly all children think in an imaginative, magical way and the nurse should be aware of this. All children need praise and rewards, but they also need to be corrected when the situation demands. Guidance must be given to each child, whether healthy or ill, but they must be allowed to express themselves and develop their own individuality.

Children have a tendency to imitate. When they do this they are not being rude, but are passing through the normal stages of a childhood.

All children in hospital must be given security and love. A sense of security can be achieved by allowing them to wear their own clothes, play with their own toys, and use the name they have at home. If every effort is made to adopt the routine the child follows at home wherever possible, and to take into consideration food fads and other idiosyncrasies, the child should feel more secure.

More hospitals are allowing parents, brothers and sisters to visit as often as they can. In most hospitals mothers are being actively encouraged to stay with their child. These are very positive ways of ensuring that the child feels loved and secure, and not isolated from the rest of the family.

Adolescents as patients

The period of adolescence is a stressful one as the adolescent goes through a period of physical, intellectual and social change. Adolescents are self-conscious of their physical appearance and are sensitive to the opinions of adults. They need time to adjust to this change.

The period of adolescence is one of insecurity and lack of confidence, although the adolescent may appear brash and full of self-confidence. This is usually a cover-up as most adolescents are sensitive, especially to the suffering of others and they become hurt easily. When adolescents are patients, illness is extremely threatening and upsetting. Ideally, adolescents should be nursed together when ill and when convalescent, as they are very supportive of each other.

Adolescents strive for independence, and since adults tend to be more rigid in their thinking they may clash with them. The adult can feel intimidated by the adolescent patient who rebels against the standards and attitudes of an older generation; the result is tension within the ward. Sometimes these patients feel more secure if nursed in single rooms, especially if they are the only adolescent patient in the ward.

Communication between adolescents and adults may be lacking, and the nursing team may not be fully aware of the difficulty which some adolescents have in expressing what they want to say. Also, adolescents are often shy, modest people who feel threatened if intimate procedures are carried out by nurses of their own age. It helps if these procedures are carried out in a matter-of-fact way, or it is better still if a mature, older nurse is available to carry out these duties.

Generally, adolescents have a lot of surplus energy and need to be kept occupied in useful activities. This can create a problem in long-stay wards such as orthopaedic wards where many patients feel well but are immobile. Imaginative thinking on the part of the nursing team to create useful occupational therapy is vital.

The elderly as patients

Elderly patients, like adolescents, are going through a time of change; they physically slow down, may become introverted and socially lack a definite role. This process of change will affect their response to, and how they cope with, being in hospital.

Elderly people often feel insecure. They sometimes have difficulty in feeling worthwhile and useful, mainly because they are becoming slower physically, but also because of a lack of stimulation, from a society which tends to reject them. This feeling is enhanced as the family grows up and becomes independent. If support from the family is lacking, the feeling of insecurity is more pronounced. The elderly patients must be encouraged to be as independent as possible, and should also be involved in decision-making relating to their care. The nurse can help by being positive. Whilst in hospital it is essential to keep the elderly active and occupied. The nurse who is able to make the patients take an interest in things around them will have alert and responsive patients.

As the body slows down physically, there may be deterioration in vision, hearing and mobility. On admission these disabilities must be watched for and allowances made for them. The elderly tend to have well-established habits and routines, and any change in their routine will create anxiety and a need for security. Encouraging patients to have photographs on lockers, to get dressed during the day, to read the newspapers, and to follow their normal eating pattern will help them to adapt to hospital. It may be difficult for an elderly patient to adapt to a new and strange environment, and nurses must appreciate this and not expect them to conform meekly to their wishes.

In the elderly, feelings can be aroused very easily and possibly excessively. They may be aggressive, stubborn, demanding or child-like. The sister or charge nurse must make sure that the nurses are aware of this. Many, but by no means all, elderly people prefer the company of their peer group rather than the younger generation, as they have common interests about which they can talk together.

As with most other patients, privacy and the preservation of dignity is extremely important to the older patient. With a little imagination and tact most nurses are able to preserve the patient's dignity, along with the provision of privacy.

When many people realize that they are ageing, faith resurges. Suggesting a visit by the spiritual adviser, or encouraging them to go to services in the hospital chapel, may be very much appreciated, but must not be forced.

If the elderly patients are given reassurance, attention, understanding, tact, sympathy and companionship, most will respond in a positive way.

Attendance at the outpatient department

The outpatient department is usually the point at which the patients and their families make their first contact with the hospital. Obviously their reception in this department is extremely important as it will effect their overall view of the hospital.

If patients are made to feel at ease by the staff in the department, they will feel less apprehensive if admission to hospital becomes necessary.

The staff in the outpatient department have an opportunity to assess the patient, and to note any previous care the community nursing service or the local authority provide for the patient at home.

If it is decided that the patient will need to be admitted to a ward at a later date the patient may be given guidance about possible length of stay, and the facilities available, such as the visiting arrangements. This will also give the patient an opportunity to obtain answers to any queries.

If there is a good relationship between the outpatient department and the ward staff it may be possible for the patient to be taken to the ward and introduced to the nurses prior to admission. Alternatively, a nurse from the ward may meet the patient in the outpatient department.

As links between outpatient clinics and the wards strengthen, there are more opportunities to enable ward nurses to attend and help organize their consultant clinics. This will help to improve the continuity of patient care, benefiting both patients and staff. It may also help the patient with his or her preparation for admission to hospital. Alternatively, outpatient department nurses may work on the appropriate ward periodically.

Some outpatient departments have specific nurses for different specialities who act as resource persons, able to guide and educate patients and colleagues and act as a contact point. The named nurse philosophy is also being extended to patients in outpatient departments.

As with medical notes, nursing records may be commenced in the outpatient department, detailing information gained about the patient which may be very relevant for the nurses planning care once the patient is admitted to the ward.

Planned admission

Patients who know they are to be admitted to hospital will have had time to think about their admission and what it means to them. They will have had an opportunity to make any necessary plans. This might involve the care of the children, transport for family visitors, informing employer, or care of the business. Some patients may want to make sure that their affairs are in order, like the elderly lady who paid her rent for a month in advance, made her will and paid all outstanding bills. It is important for patients to be given this opportunity, and it is essential that, prior to admission, patients have an indication of the possible length of stay and what is involved for them. Information sent out by the hospital should tell patients what to bring with them.

The sister or charge nurse should ensure that the nurse or nurses who will be caring for the patients are aware of their expected arrival. The nurse should welcome them by name, introducing herself or himself, the nurse or nurses who will look after the patient, and the patients in the beds nearby. It often happens that a bed is not immediately available for the patient. A brief explanation to the patient and his or her relatives will help to allay anxiety. If it is possible the patient and relatives should be sat in a comfortable area and given a cup of tea. Even if harassed, the nurse should never show her or his irritation or harassment if there is likely to be a problem finding a bed. It is not the patient's fault. Ways of reducing anxiety are discussed earlier (pp. 142–5).

Patients are usually sociable and friendly once they have got over their initial shyness and anxiety, and they tend to create a pleasant atmosphere and boost each other's morale. However, if the nurse admitting the patient is abrupt or offhand this will make it much more difficult for the patient to settle.

Certain standard particulars are required from each patient on admission, and will be entered on the patient's nursing records. These particulars should include:

- Registration number
- Name
- Address
- Telephone number
- Date of birth
- Marital status
- Occupation
- Religion
- Name and address of next of kin or person to be contacted; legally this does not have to be a relative but a person named by the patient
- Telephone number to contact relatives; to avoid confusion a note should be made of the owner of the telephone, the relationship to the patient, and the times that the telephone number is available
- Name and address of general practitioner, district nurse and social services
- Consultant
- Diagnosis – nursing and medical
- Time of admission
- Ward
- Hospital.

These details need to be checked with the patient, or person accompanying the patient, and not copied straight from the admission slip or old case notes.

Other information may be required at or during admission.

On admission, each patient should have an identification bracelet attached, giving his or her full name and registration number, and any other information required by the hospital.

Many patients bring drugs with them. The doctor will need to see these and they must be stored in a safe place, either on the ward or in the pharmacy depending on the policy of the hospital, or given to the patient's relatives to take home. They should never be disposed of without the patient's permission as they are the property of the patient.

Case notes and X-rays are usually sent to the ward prior to admission. Ward clerks or secretaries may be part of the ward team and will be responsible for obtaining these. In wards where there is no clerical assistance this task is usually carried out by the nurse admitting the patient. Case notes are usually obtained through the consultant's secretary in the medical records department.

At the time of admission, certain physiological measurements such as temperature, pulse rate, respiratory rate, blood pressure, weight and height will be measured by the nurse. These will be determined by the patient's clinical condition and diagnosis.

Once the nurse has taken the baseline observations, the doctor is informed that the patient is in the ward. In some situations the ward doctor may always see the waiting list patients at a set time, such as in the afternoon following admission that morning. The nurses should be aware of these arrangements so as to be able to inform their patients.

Emergency admission

The patient who is admitted as an emergency will have had little or no time to prepare for hospitalization, and will be frightened, bewildered and often very ill. The importance of the patient's first contact with the nursing team, both in the accident and emergency department and in the ward, cannot be over emphasized.

Once in the ward, the patient is helped to be as comfortable as possible, and any immediate nursing intervention indicated, such as maintenance of a clear airway in an unconscious patient, is instigated. The patient is admitted by the nurse concerned and relevant physiological measurements taken and recorded. It is wise to inform the doctor of the patient's arrival on the ward as soon as possible, but the timing of this will depend on the clinical condition of the patient.

Obtaining and checking relevant information, provision of identification bracelet and care of any drugs brought in by the patient are dealt with in the same way as for the patient admitted from the waiting list.

It is important that the patient's district nurses and social services are informed of the admission, to avoid causing unnecessary visits and anxiety.

Informing relatives and friends

Patients admitted from the waiting list are usually accompanied by a relative or a friend. If not, it should be confirmed with the patients that their relatives know of their admission. In exceptional circumstances it may be the patient's wish that the relatives are not informed. This wish should be respected but clearly stated in the nursing records.

When a relative accompanies the patient, the sister, charge nurse or nurse caring for the patient should see the relative and give information such as:

- Visiting times
- The most convenient time to telephone
- Possible length of stay
- Date of operation or specific investigations
- Anything the patient may need
- Anything the patient may not be allowed, for example, certain foods.

In some hospitals, patients' relatives are asked to take indoor clothes home but it is becoming more common for patients to be allowed to dress in their day clothes. The relatives may also be asked to take the patient's drugs home.

When a patient is admitted to hospital in an emergency and the relatives do not know, they must be notified straightaway. However, if the patient is fully alert and over 16 years of age the patient's permission should be obtained first. The patient may not wish anyone to be notified of his or her admission. In this case it is imperative that this request is fully recorded in the nursing notes. Whether it is the responsibility of the casualty department staff or the ward staff to contact relatives will depend on the policy of the hospital.

Contacting a patient's relatives may be done by telephone, telephone message to a neighbour or place of work if known, or by police message. A police message is sent by contacting the nearest police station, which can be located through the hospital switchboard, the telephone directory or through the police headquarters for the metropolitan district or county concerned. Police personnel are usually most cooperative in this matter, and will contact the ward once the message has been delivered.

If there are no known relatives and the patient is able to state this, this is recorded clearly in the nursing records. If the patient is confused or unconscious a number of sources may be pursued in an attempt to confirm this, such as the patient's general practitioner, neighbours or friends. If all else fails the police can be approached.

Relatives may be asked to give information in certain circumstances, as with a child or a confused or unconscious patient. Other information from relatives might include medical and social background, drugs currently being taken, and so forth. In the case of a child, food fads and the name by which the child is usually called are always required. If a patient is aphasic or dysphasic a simple detail such as whether the patient takes sugar in tea is of great importance to the patient. Written consent from relatives for operation or certain procedures may also be required in the case of a minor, a confused patient or an unconscious patient.

In these situations it is advisable to ask the relatives to wait until the doctor has examined the patient so that the doctor may obtain any facts or information which the patient is not able to give.

Clothing and personal belongings

Depending on local policy the nurse may or may not be expected to list the patient's items of clothing and personal belongings. Common practice in most general hospitals is that patients are allowed to keep their clothes. This may not be the practice in psychiatric and elderly care units. Patients who retain their clothes, jewellery, etc., should be aware that they are responsible for them. It is wise to advise patients to have valuable jewellery and large amounts of money taken home or put into the hospital safe. The procedure for the safe custody of valuables in hospital will include obtaining signatures from the patient and two nurses, and giving the patient a receipt. The valuables are either taken to the hospital cashier or, at night and at weekends, to the person in charge of the hospital. When valuables are taken for safe-keeping this should always be recorded in the nursing records.

If a patient is unconscious and money or jewellery is given to his or her relative, it is usual for a signature to be obtained from the relative. In many hospitals this responsibility will lie with the hospital cashier or the administrator's department, but in some hospitals it may be carried out by the senior nurse on duty in the ward.

Other patients

Private

The *private patient* pays the consultant and the hospital for all treatment received. The number of private patients allowed at any one time is limited. The beds are allocated nationally on an area basis and are booked through one central point by the admissions controller, the consultant or the consultant's secretary. Patients are only able to be booked in if a private bed is free. The health authority is not allowed to have more private patients than the beds allocated for that purpose.

Amenity

The *amenity patient* is a patient who prefers the privacy of a single room, for which a fee is charged, but receives treatment through the National Health Service. The patient must understand that if this room is required for another patient for medical reasons, the room has to be vacated.

Courtesy

The term *courtesy patient* is usually reserved for a member of staff who is given a single room if one is available, but no charge is made for it.

Service patients admitted to National Health Service hospitals

The term *Service patients* applies to full-time members of the Royal Navy, Royal Marines, Army and Royal Air Force, members of the Territorial Army and other Reserve Forces whilst undergoing training, and members of the armed services of foreign countries on loan or attached to services in the United Kingdom.

When a Service patient is admitted the responsible Service authorities must be notified immediately otherwise the patient will be classed as absent-without-leave. There are official documents for this purpose so it is essential that the ward sister or charge nurse informs the medical records officer, the administrator or the admissions officer.

The same ruling applies in the case of the death of a Service patient. When a Service patient dies, the disposal of the patient's personal effects is the responsibility of the Service authorities.

When discharged from hospital, the Service patient is normally instructed to report to his or her unit or ship and not to go directly home, unless otherwise instructed by the Service authority.

Topics for discussion

1. Patients' reactions to hospital admission.

Mrs Palm, a 72-year-old housewife was admitted to a Care of the Elderly assessment unit for investigation of increasing dyspnoea. On admission, all her clothes and unnecessary belongings were sent home. The reason given was that on this type of unit, patients sometimes had difficulty maintaining responsibility for their own possessions and that staff could not do so.

Discuss the psychological effect this action could have on the patient.

Could this practice affect the medical or nursing assessment of the patient.

Discuss alternative solutions to the problems of personal property in acute elderly care.

2. The effect of misinformation.

Mrs Elm is going to receive cerebral irradiation. On admission to the radio-therapy ward she is told by the nurse that prior to commencing radiotherapy, she will have her head shaved. This information is incorrect: Mrs Elm's hair will fall out due to the effects of the treatment, but not immediately, and she will not be required to shave her head. A wig will be fitted to match her own hair colour and style before hair loss begins.

Discuss the effects that the giving of misinformation would have on Mrs Elm. How would it affect her relationships with nursing staff in the future?

References and Suggested Reading

Abdellah, F.G. & Levine, E. (1957) Developing a measure of patient and personnel satisfaction with nursing care. *Nursing Research* 5: 10 Feb.

Barrett, J., Gessner, B.A. & Phelps, C. (1975) *The Head Nurse.* Appleton–Century–Crofts, New York.

Bennett, G. (1979) *Patients and their Doctors.* Baillière Tindall, London.

Boore, J. (1978) *Prescription for Recovery.* Churchill Livingstone/Royal College of Nursing.

Cartwright, A. (1964) *Human Relations and Hospital Care,* Institute of Community Studies, Routledge & Kegan Paul, London.

Franklin, B.L. (1974) *Patient Anxiety on Admission to Hospital.* Royal College of Nursing, London.

Hamilton Smith, S. (1972) *Nil by Mouth?* Royal College of Nursing, London.

Hayward, J. (1975) *Information – a Prescription Against Pain.* Royal College of Nursing, London.

Health Service Management – *Treatment of Service Patients in NHS Hospitals.* DHSS, HN (80)26.

Towell, D. (1975) *Understanding Psychiatric Nursing.* Royal College of Nursing, London.

Wilson-Barnett, J. (1978) In hospital: patients' feelings and opinions. *Nursing Times Occasional Paper* 74, 9 March 23: 33–34.

Wilson-Barnett, J. (1979) *Stress in Hospital – Patients' Psychological Reactions to Illness and Health Care.* Churchill Livingstone, London.

Chapter 8
The multidisciplinary team approach

The ward sister or charge nurse who is fully committed to an individual approach to patients and to giving total patient care must recognize that a team approach is necessary, and must be willing to cooperate with all other members of the health care team. Total care of patients should be the objective of every health professional, each one bringing her or his unique expertise to the team. If several health care workers are involved in the care of the patient there should be a better choice of solutions to many of the problems encountered (Fig 8.1).

A high standard of patient care depends on meeting the patients' physical, psychological and spiritual needs. No one person can do this alone, it is a team responsibility. Several health care workers may be involved in the care of one patient. These may include the ward sister or charge nurse and the nursing team, the consultant and the medical team,

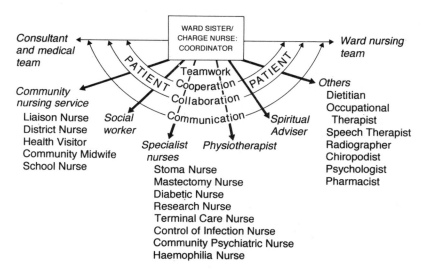

Fig. 8.1 The multidisciplinary team.

the community nursing service, specialist nurses, physiotherapist, social worker, spiritual adviser, occupational therapist, dietician, psychologist, pharmacist and therapeutic radiographer.

Each member of the team must be aware of the contribution and role of the others. The sister or charge nurse is one of the persons having frequent contact with the patient and family and may be the focal point for information about individual patients, and therefore in the best position to coordinate the multidisciplinary team. With the evolution of patient allocation and the transition to primary nursing, the primary nurse may be the coordinator. On the other hand, it could be another member of the multidisciplinary team, depending on each individual case. This means that there must be frequent contact with all other health care workers. The coordinator of the team must be approachable, must make early and appropriate referrals to other team members, and must be able to communicate effectively, giving up-to-date information and then standing back and allowing the specialists to set their own priorities. It must be emphasized here that it is of vital importance that patients and their relatives are involved in the decision-making. This is not the prerogative of the multidisciplinary team.

The concept of a multidisciplinary team approach to patient care has developed further in some hospitals than in others. In many psychiatric and care of the elderly units there seems to be a greater awareness of the need to involve other health care professionals along with nurses and doctors. Unfortunately this concept may be less obvious in many acute hospitals. In many wards the consultant still feels the need to control all aspects of patient care and is unwilling to communicate effectively with other members of the team. Some ward sisters or charge nurses take the attitude that they alone are responsible for the total care of the patient together with the consultant. The patient suffers when these attitudes prevail. For example, if the doctor insists on discharging a patient before adequate arrangements can be made at home, the patient's condition, once home, may deteriorate rapidly, resulting in readmission to hospital. The ward sister or charge nurse, social worker, district nurse or community psychiatric nurse, and possibly the physiotherapist need to be involved in this decision.

If importance is given to teamwork in patient care and the cooperation of other health care workers is obtained, limited staff resources are used more efficiently and effectively, but it is essential that all the team members communicate, collaborate and cooperate with each other. This relationship may take a long time to develop, and it is up to each member of the team to make the necessary effort.

On being appointed the sister or charge nurse must arrange to meet and get to know the health care workers involved in the care of the patients on the ward. If a relationship of trust and respect is built up this will assist communication and cooperation. Each person must be willing to see the points of view of the others, and the sister or charge nurse needs to understand and respect the role of the other members and their expectations of the person in charge of the ward. They too need to know what the sister or charge nurse expects of them. Once a good working relationship is built up this will become apparent, as long as there is good will and cooperation on both sides.

The ward sister or charge nurse will need to demonstrate tact and diplomacy, as the job involves relating to different types of people from various disciplines, each with specific ideals and skills. It must be remembered that the sister or charge nurse is usually one of the few stable forces in the multidisciplinary team. Other members, such as the house officer or the physiotherapist, may change at frequent intervals.

A commitment to patient-centred nursing enables nurses at the bed-side to be in touch with other health care workers, and to communicate freely with them about the patient's total needs. In order that this involvement develops further the sister or charge nurse must be seen by all the ward nurses to be positive about the team approach, and about involving others.

The ward nurse is an influential member of the patient care team. As a result many other health care workers especially the social worker, community nurses and the spiritual adviser, who are often dependent on the nurse for their initial contact with the patients, rely on her or him for much of their information. They see themselves as visitors to the ward and will need to feel welcome.

By being pleasant and approachable, the nurse will help and encourage other health care workers such as the social worker or spiritual adviser. There must also be a willingness to communicate with them and to share relevant information when indicated, for example, it is usually important for the social worker to know something of the patient's background. Early referrals will enable other members of the team to work as effectively as possible. Referrals need to be appropriate so the nurse will need to have full knowledge of the role of the other team members.

A sensitivity to the needs of the patients and their relatives must be shown so that an assessment can be made whether to refer either the patient or the relatives to another member of the health team.

Fifty-one-year-old Mrs Elder, married but with no children, was admitted to hospital in the terminal stages of her illness. Her two regular visitors were her husband and her elderly mother. Her husband had been referred to the social worker who, it was felt, could provide support for him in her counselling role.

The ward sister then had a long talk with Mrs Elder's mother who was extremely distressed as she was very close to her daughter. She had another daughter who lived 200 miles away and was severely disabled with multiple sclerosis. Mrs Elder's mother had also lost her husband two years previously. The ward sister felt that the patient's mother also needed a great deal of support and someone who could spend time with her, especially when Mrs Elder eventually died, so she referred her to the social worker. The social worker spent much time with both Mr Elder and his mother-in-law before Mrs Elder's death, and after her death was able to visit them both in their homes and help them through the stages of bereavement which they both found extremely bewildering and difficult. If the ward sister had not assessed the need of the mother in this situation it may well have been that the husband received help and support but that the mother was left to cope alone.

Mrs Tamarind, a young Jamaican mother of three, was dying in hospital after a short illness. Her husband was extremely distressed, wanting to do all that he could for his wife. The ward sister spent a lot of time talking to Mr Tamarind, and tentatively suggested that if he agreed, she could ask the spiritual adviser to come to talk to him. He readily accepted the offer and the sister contacted the spiritual adviser straightaway. He came immediately and spent a long time with Mrs and Mrs Tamarind. They both received much comfort from this visit.

The role of each health care worker is complementary to the other. They may overlap and will sometimes be interchangeable, depending on the nature of the ward. It is necessary for the nurse in charge of the ward to be aware of:

(1)   The role and functions of each health care worker
(2)   The policy for referring patients and recording the referrals.

The consultant and the medical team

The consultants are extremely influential members of the health care team by virtue of their concept of clinical responsibility and their influence on other groups. The consultant has, however, the authority to delegate aspects of care to the other team members, as long as those team members are competent. The team members are responsible for their own actions.

The doctors make the clinical decisions affecting the patients as they have the necessary training and knowledge. These decisions are usually made at the ward round, so it is not essential that the doctors are present at other team meetings although it is a good idea to have the medical staff represented if possible.

The relationship between the nurse in charge of the ward and the doctors is important, as they spend a lot of time together, and many decisions should be joint nursing and medical decisions. The ward sister or charge nurse, however, must stand firm when necessary, as there are some doctors who will try to tell her or him how to nurse the patients. Nursing decisions and prescribing nursing care should be carried out by the nursing team. Florence Nightingale said in 1867: 'don't let the doctor make himself Head Nurse.' This is still sound advice today.

Ward rounds

Ward rounds are usually held at set times through the week and it is important that all nursing staff know when they are held.

It is not necessary for the ward sister or charge nurse to arrange her or his days off around ward rounds, as this might lead to a situation where the consultant is not willing to do a ward round with any other nurse, or if doing so, makes it very unpleasant for the nurse by not listening to her or his contribution and being highly critical. The duty rota should be planned so that the staff nurse does some of the ward rounds, and not only when the sister or charge nurse is on holiday. With a primary nursing organization, it will be the primary nurse's function to liaise with medical colleagues concerning the patients for whom she or he is responsible.

It is of educational benefit for the sister or charge nurse to take staff nurses, enrolled nurses and student nurses on consultants' ward rounds. This will give them an opportunity to take part in discussion relating to the patients they are caring for and it will give them an insight into how ward rounds are conducted, giving them more confidence to discuss patients with doctors and other health care workers.

Staff nurses, enrolled nurses or student nurses are all capable of accompanying the house officer or registrar when the sister or charge nurse is on duty; this is most meaningful if the nurse allocated to the patient is involved. It is, however, essential that an opportunity is given for the nurse to report back to the nursing team.

Patients' case notes and X-rays will be required for the ward round and it is the responsibility of the ward clerk or secretary to make sure that notes and X-rays are available. Some wards, however, are not fortunate enough to have clerical help, and therefore the preparation of notes and X-rays becomes the responsibility of the ward sister or charge nurse, or of the doctor.

Certain equipment will also need to be at hand, depending on the type of ward. On an orthopaedic ward an X-ray viewing box is essential. On a medical ward round sphygmomanometer, ophthalmoscope, auroscope and central nervous system examination tray with tuning fork, patella hammer, cotton wool, pins and equipment required to test the sensory nerves will be needed. On an ENT ward auroscope and headmirror will be required.

If the consultant believes in total care of the patients, he or she will accept that no one person can meet all the patients' needs but that this is a team response. If this is his or her philosophy it will probably be the practice to include other health care workers such as the community liaison nurse, social worker, physiotherapist or radiographer on the ward round.

Any decisions made on the ward round, such as special investigations to be arranged, date of operation, date of discharge or transfer, should all be noted by the sister or charge nurse or the patient's nurse and the appropriate action taken on completion of the round.

The community nursing service

The community nursing service includes district nurses, health visitors, district midwives, school nurses, practice nurses and community psychiatric nurses. Liaison between hospital and any one of these services will vary from hospital to hospital, but referrals should be made by a nurse. In some hospitals there will be a liaison district nurse or health visitor who will take all referrals from the wards and departments and then liaise with the appropriate district nurse or health visitor in the community.

District nurse

The district nurse is able to give skilled nursing care to all persons living in the community. These skills are varied and include general care, bathing, changing dressings, removal of stitches and clips, injections, catheterizations and any nursing care that was given to the patient in hospital and considered necessary following discharge home, as long as the care can be adapted to the home situation. The district nurse is also involved in teaching and educating the patient and the family and can play a major part in providing support and comfort for patients with life-threatening illnesses or who are terminally ill, and their families.

One example of specific care is the supervision of nasogastric feeding. The district nurse may be asked to assess the ability of the relatives to do this, then educate them to assist with or give the feeds, even though this will have begun on the ward prior to the patient's discharge. The district nurse may visit three or four times a day until she or he is happy that the patient's relatives are able to cope. Another example of her or his care is supporting the new diabetic who is faced with giving injections for the first time at home.

In some towns and cities the community nursing service provide a 24-hour operation with the provision of a night nursing team. This service varies from a nursing auxiliary staying in the patient's home all night to a visiting service. The benefit gained by the auxiliary staying all night is that the patient's relatives are able to get a night's rest. The auxiliary takes the place of a relative and is supported by visits from the night sister.

The decision to refer a patient to the district nursing service is a nursing decision which is made by the ward sister or charge nurse or the nurse caring for the patient following discussion with the ward sister or charge nurse, and the referral is a nurse to nurse referral. Whenever a verbal referral is made, this is always followed up by a referral letter, or a copy of the nursing records, and the fact that the patient has been referred to the district nurse is documented in the patient's nursing records.

Health visitor

The health visitor has a responsibility to the whole family, although the first priority is child health care. The health visitor is trained to recognize problems which may result in either illness or breakdown of the family unit. A good example is non-accidental injury to the very young or the elderly.

The health visitor is concerned with the prevention or early detection of illness, providing support during times of stress and arranging the services of other agencies when indicated. A large part of the work is concerned with health education.

The decision to refer a patient to the health visitor is usually a nursing one but may be taken in conjunction with the liaison health visitor if available, or alternatively, with the liaison district nurse or the social worker.

Community midwife

The community midwife provides antenatal and postnatal care, attending confinements at home and also in hospital in many instances. When mothers are discharged from hospital the midwife becomes responsible for their care until this is taken over by the health visitor. Many midwives are now becoming involved in genetic counselling and family planning.

School nurse

In certain areas the function is a combined health visitor/school nurse one, and referrals are made via the health visitor; but in other instances the school service is separate to the health visitor service. There is, however, close liaison between the two disciplines. The school nurse assists with the medical examination of all children, and may also provide certain treatment for the children. If it is necessary for treatment to continue over the weekend the school nurse liaises with the district nurse to give treatment at home.The school nurse also makes home visits as required.

The school nurse may work in a special school such as schools for the blind or deaf or for the mentally or physically handicapped.

Practice nurse

The role of the practice nurse is rapidly developing, particularly in practices where General Practitioners manage their own budgets. Practice nurses work within a general practitioner practice, employed by the doctors. They may be responsible for a wide range of activities from family planning to Well Woman or Well Man health checks and screening. They also remove sutures and do minor dressings.

When referring patients to any of the community nursing services the following information is required:

- Name
- Age
- Address
- Next of kin
- General practitioner's name and address
- Diagnosis and whether patient and his or her relatives are aware of the diagnosis and prognosis
- Hospital consultant
- Treatment in hospital
- Treatment and care required at home
- Date treatment is to commence
- Social background
- Any other relevant information.

When a referral is made it is recorded in the patient's nursing records and a referral letter is completed and either sent by post, or given to the patient or his or her relatives to give to the community nurse concerned (Table 8.1).

Table 8.1 Functions of community nurses and methods of referral.

Functions	Methods of referral
District nurse	Hospital/community liaison nurse
Skilled nursing care	District nurse via general practitioner's surgery or health
General care	centre
Bathing	Designated central point of contact in the community
Dressings	nursing service – this is usually a nurse manager or a
Injections	secretary
Catheterizations	Handbook of Community Nursing (the health authority in
Specific nursing care	which the patient resides must be known and the
Assessment of patient and	Handbook will give the health district, the main towns
relatives	and areas served and the contact point)
Advising patient and relatives	
Supervising patient and	
relatives	
Supporting and counselling	
patient and relatives	
Educating patient and	
relatives	
Night nursing service	
Health visitor	
Promotion of health	Hospital/community liaison health visitor
Prevention of ill-health	Designated central point of contact in the community
Advising	nursing service
Educating	General practitioner's surgery or the health centre
Supporting	
Enlisting other agencies	
Community midwife	
Antenatal care	Community midwifery service
Postnatal care	
Home and hospital deliveries	
Family planning	
Genetic counselling	
School nurse	
Health surveillance of school	As for health visitor
children	
Health education of school	
children	
Regular screening tests e.g.	
hearing, vision	
Work in special schools e.g.	
for maladjusted children	
Treatment for school	
children e.g. dressings,	
injections	

Hospital social workers

All social workers are employed by the local authority, even if based at hospitals. Some social workers are attached to consultant's units, others are ward based. The work of the social worker is varied but the role of the social worker in hospital is to help patients and their families with the stresses that arise from, or may have contributed to their illness and which may impede recovery. This covers a wide spectrum from counselling patients about personal problems to making practical arrangements for aftercare. This requires a versatile approach.

If hospital social workers are to be effective members of the health care team early referral to them is essential.

Referrals can be made by nurses, doctors, other disciplines, the patients themselves or patients' relatives. However, it is usually ward sisters or charge nurses who make most referrals so they must fully understand the social worker's role to be able to refer appropriately. The sister or charge nurse should be prepared to use the expertise of the social workers, allowing them to become involved with the patient at ward level. Communication between sisters or charge nurses and social workers must be good, and this is based on their getting to know each other as people, and developing a sense of trust in each other. The ward sister or charge nurse can make it very difficult for the social workers to do their job by withholding referrals and necessary information such as particulars of a patient's background, and even excluding the social worker altogether. The building up of a good relationship between the sister or charge nurse and the social worker is vital to the patient's well-being.

For this to happen, however, social workers have to be aware of ward sisters' or charge nurses' expectations of them. This will include being available when needed, though this may not always be possible given other commitments, informing the ward sister or charge nurse of plans made or action taken, such as arranging convalescence or home help, and passing on relevant information when counselling patients or their relatives.

Nurses in the ward team will take their lead from the ward sister or charge nurse. If great importance is attached to the input of the social worker the nurses will do likewise. One way of enabling staff nurses and enrolled nurses to be more aware of the functions of the social worker is to arrange for them to spend one or two days with a social worker. This will also help to foster good relationships.

The social workers have much information readily available to help the patient. Therefore, if in any doubt the patient should be referred to the social worker. It is important that the social workers are involved with outpatients as well as inpatients.

The main functions of the social worker are to:

(1) Assess the needs, difficulties and problems of the patient and relatives.
(2) Counsel and support both patients and relatives.
(3) In relation to the needs mobilize the resources available through the local authority social services department.
(4) Act as liaison with all voluntary agencies and other services, for example, housing department, Department of Social Security.

Assessing the needs

The social worker is trained to assess the individual's needs and act appropriately. This involves taking into account all aspects of the patient's personality and way of life, and relationships with relatives. Understanding these, the social worker then plans with the patient, and family if possible, how best to help and this may be continued for as long as the social worker feels it is necessary.

Counselling and support

The social worker is someone to whom patients can relate when in hospital and discuss problems which may have no direct relationship with their illness. Often patients feel unable to discuss these sort of problems with nursing or medical staff. If very ill or dying patients appear worried, they may be worrying about their relatives, so it is important to involve the social worker immediately.

The social worker is able to counsel and provide support for patient's relatives, especially the relatives of the terminally ill. The social workers are one of the few groups of hospital personnel who are able to follow up patients or relatives at home. Therefore, they are able to provide support for bereaved relatives during the grieving period. Many nurses are unaware of this area of the social workers' role and so many vital referrals are missed. For example, it might be felt that it is not necessary to refer the wealthy businessman whose wife is dying, as the social worker is seen as being associated with arranging practical aspects of care. This man, however, will need as much support as is available during the period of bereavement.

Mobilizing resources available

As social workers are employed by the local authority they have direct access to many resources provided by the authority:

- Home help and home wardens
- Residential accommodation for the elderly, mentally handicapped, mentally ill and physically handicapped
- Day centres for elderly, mentally and physically handicapped
- Temporary and long-term foster placements for children
- Practical help, aids and adaptations such as ramps and bath seats, plus many facilities for specifically handicapped groups.

Liaising with voluntary organizations and other services

It is the job of the social worker to put the patient in touch with any other agencies whose facilities will help the patient. The social worker represents the patient, seeing that the patient receives the optimum help available. In some hospitals this includes arranging convalescence.

There are a variety of associations which may offer counselling, support or practical help for patients and their families. Some of these operate purely at a national level, while others are national associations with many local branches. Examples of these are Cruse (national organization for counselling and support of the widowed and their children) and the Mastectomy Association. There may also be organizations which are run by the local community such as good neighbour schemes, church clubs and clubs for people with specific disabilities such as Alzheimer's disease. The social worker should be aware of the facilities available, both nationally and locally, and is in a good position to make the information about how to contact them available to patients and their relatives. Some useful names and addresses can be found in Appendix II.

Appropriate benefits and financial assistance can be obtained for patients and their relatives through the Department of Social Security. These include supplementary benefits, family income supplement, attendance allowance, disability living allowance and the national insurance death grant.

The earlier a referral is made, the sooner the relationship between the social worker and the patient can be established. So that referrals are not overlooked and in order that the liaison between the ward nursing team and the social workers is made as strong as possible, it could be suggested to the social workers that they visit the ward at set times during the week, and also attend the ward handovers whenever possible.

Specialist nurses or clinical nurse specialists

Nurses are beginning to specialize in different aspects of care, specialist nurses or clinical nurse specialists being available to advise and assist both patients and ward staff. Nurses in the past have been reluctant to call on the expertise of their colleagues, but no nurse can know all there is to know about every nursing speciality today.

Specialist nurses may be sisters or charge nurses who have had much experience in a certain field of nursing, possibly having completed a course. They may be hospital or district based and may have some input into the community nursing service, visiting patients in their own homes. Others stay in their own wards or departments and act as advisers to others. On the other hand, the specialist nurse may have very specialized knowledge and clinical expertise, and be directly responsible to the employing authority, working in close liaison with other nurses and also doctors. They are consulted by reason of their expertise, advising on patient care and formulating nursing plans, teaching and carrying out research projects. In some areas they may be involved in the direct care of a small selected group of patients. Specialist nurses, regardless of their speciality, need to have a clinical, managerial, educational and research component within their role (RCN, 1988).

Not all hospitals, however, have the service of specialist nurses but when available it may include such specialities as diabetes, haemophilia, research, terminal care, control of infection, stoma care and mastectomy care. The community psychiatric nurse also comes into this category. The extent of their responsibility will vary from one health district to another and the sister or charge nurse should ensure that she or he is aware of the availability of specialist nurses, the extent of their responsibility and methods of referral.

There are many advantages to both patients and nurses if knowledge and expertise such as this is readily available. It is a post, however, which must be interpreted with great tact and diplomacy so that the role of the specialist nurse does not erode that of the ward sister or charge nurse.

Physiotherapists

The physiotherapist is a vital member of the health care team in most wards. The physiotherapist's functions are varied and include:

- Chest physiotherapy
    general chest care
    pre- and postoperative care
- Mobilization and rehabilitation
    re-education of movement
    long-term advice and support

home assessments
advising the static patient
- Specific care
hand and orthopaedic treatment
heat treatment
diathermy.

The general role of the physiotherapist is that of advising and teaching the patient. This sometimes includes patients' relatives and nurses on such subjects as the best methods of lifting disabled patients. The physiotherapist cooperates with the other health care workers in the team and liaises with them when planning the treatment schedules for patient care. The effectiveness of the care given by the physiotherapist is based on building up good relationships within the team and developing effective working arrangements with the consultant and ward nurses. Good communication is therefore of paramount importance.

In most hospitals a physiotherapist is on call in the evenings and at the weekends and there will be a specific procedure laid down for contacting the physiotherapist.

Spiritual adviser

Some hospital spiritual advisers are full-time workers, others part-time, therefore the amount of time they are able to spend at the hospital will help to determine their involvement. Many who work part-time in the hospital are only allocated three or four hours per week there although many of them attend for much longer than this. Many nurses are unaware of the limited time that some hospital spiritual advisers can be in the hospital. However, some hospitals have lay persons who act as assistants to the spiritual adviser.

Although other members of the hospital team have close contact with the spiritual adviser it is often the ward sister or charge nurse who links him or her with the patient. It is usually the nurse who uses her or his initiative and suggests that the spiritual adviser visits a certain patient or his or her relative or suggests to the patient or relative that the spiritual adviser is a person who might be able to provide support and help at a difficult time.

Mrs Willow, a lady of 43 years with a serious illness, was very frightened of dying. However, she felt guilty that she was so frightened as she was a Roman Catholic. She talked to the ward sister about her fear and her feelings of guilt. The ward sister was able to speak to the Roman Catholic priest who then went to see Mrs Willow. He talked for a long time with her and was able to rationalize her fears and her guilt and help her to get her feelings into perspective. If the ward sister had not brought up the subject with the spiritual adviser Mrs Willow probably never would have, and would have spent the remainder of her life feeling guilty.

Many nurses think that the seriously ill or dying are the only patients who require the support of the spiritual adviser. The spiritual adviser, however, can help and support patients who are bewildered and frightened and need someone to talk to whom they can trust, but who is not medically or emotionally involved. Other patients who may be referred to the spiritual adviser are patients who have lost their sight, lonely patients, long-stay patients, patients who know they have cancer, patients showing signs of stress, and those who have to make decisions which will affect their lives and that of their families.

The spiritual adviser may also be of valuable support to those patients admitted because of attempted suicide, the very ill, the dying, patients who are bereaved or mothers who have lost their babies.

Relatives have a need for counselling, comfort, support and companionship and are shocked by sudden deterioration of a loved one, accident, myocardial infarction or any bad news. The relatives are often left alone whilst all the ward staff are with the patient during a crisis. The spiritual adviser, if made aware of the situation, is usually willing to talk to the patient's relatives and bring objectivity into such situations. It also gives the relatives an opportunity to freely express their emotions.

Members of the nursing staff can often be helped by the spiritual adviser. Pain, suffering and death cause stress for the staff who themselves need support, rather than protection, in these situations. The spiritual adviser, a member of the caring team, can help nurses get their feelings, fears and anger into perspective. Following stressful emergency situations when some nurses may be distraught, the sister or charge nurse can involve the spiritual adviser in discussion with the ward team – problem sharing reduces stress.

So that the spiritual adviser is seen as a member of the ward team rather than a visitor, it will be helpful if the ward sister or charge nurse demonstrates a positive, friendly approach, asking for advice and specific help as required. By doing this she or he will convey to the nursing team that the spiritual adviser is an important member of the multidisciplinary team. The spiritual adviser depends largely on the nurse in charge of the ward for direction to the appropriate place at the right time.

Other members of the multidisciplinary team

Dietician

The dietician is usually more involved in wards where patients need special diets. This will include wards such as renal units, diabetic units and metabolic units. The dietician, however, is also available to advise and teach not only patients needing special diets but also those who need general dietetic guidance.

When patients are not able to tolerate ordinary meals the nurse will need to liaise with the dietician in order to obtain alternatives for the patient. Consideration will need to be given to what the patient is able to have, what the patient can cope with, what the patient likes and dislikes and also what is available. In some hospitals the catering manager will be the person with whom the nurse will discuss such problems.

Occupational therapist

Occupational therapists are more likely to be available in specialist units such as care of the elderly and psychiatric units and stroke rehabilitation units rather than in the general hospitals. They provide diversional therapy for patients and are also involved in rehabilitation and retraining. This will include teaching disabled patients to dress, cook and regain their independence. Diversional therapy may be indicated for chronically ill patients and those patients who are in the preterminal phase of their illness, e.g. the patient with cancer. The occupational therapist will also train the physically and the mentally disabled to adapt to their limitations. It is usual for the patient to attend the occupational therapy department if well enough.

During the rehabilitation process of the physically disabled the occupational therapist, together with the physiotherapist, will carry out an assessment of the patient in the patient's home and make suggestions for making appropriate adaptations. When a home visit is arranged it is suggested that a nurse from the ward also accompanies the patient in an attempt to meet the patient's total needs.

Speech therapist

Speech therapists see both inpatients and outpatients, referrals being made by the doctor or the nurse. Their work is educational and rehabilitative.

Patients who are referred include those who have speech defects due to a congenital disability, trauma – either accidental or following surgery

– and patients who have had a laryngectomy or a cerebrovascular accident. The patients may be seen by the speech therapist either in the ward or in the outpatient department. It is wise to include the speech therapist in multidisciplinary team meetings when indicated.

Radiographer

Although the diagnostic radiographers will be involved in the investigation of many patients, this is usually at departmental level.

Therapeutic radiographers are involved in the treatment of patients in their department but may be involved in ward rounds and multidisciplinary team discussions about the patients. Their involvement is very important as they, too, may be treating the patients over a long period of time and have day-to-day contact with them, giving them an opportunity to discuss with the patients their treatment, their progress and their anxieties. It is essential that the radiographer is able to discuss these aspects with the rest of the team.

Multidisciplinary team meetings

Although the ideal situation is one in which all the health care workers meet together on a regular basis this will not always be possible especially if one or more of the team members refuses to cooperate. Meetings can, however, be started in a small way, with the social worker and physiotherapist being invited to meet the ward sister or charge nurse on the ward at weekly intervals to discuss problems related to the care of the patients.

Another way of involving other members of the team is to invite one or two to the ward report on a certain day each week. This opportunity is usually welcomed by the social worker, spiritual adviser or physiotherapist. The house office or registrar might be willing to participate, giving the nursing team the chance to discuss particular problems with them. In the case of the social worker it gives her or him the opportunity to select those patients who she or he feels best able to help. Different health care workers can be invited to join at intervals until a full multidisciplinary team meeting is held regularly.

Alternatively, the sister or charge nurse can suggest to the consultant that other members be invited along to discuss particular patients over a cup of coffee before or after the ward round. This gives an opportunity for everyone to become involved in the care of the patient and understand the involvement of the other team members.

The relationship of each team member to the patient will be very different, and the contributions of each will vary from time to time. It must also be accepted that there will be an overlap of functions in many instances and the difference between the role of each may sometimes be blurred. For example, the ward sister or charge nurse may make all the arrangements for one patient to be discharged home, whereas in the case of another patient this may become the responsibility of the social worker. Each team member's involvement in patient counselling will vary from patient to patient as it is not the sole responsibility of any one person.

When the multidisciplinary team meets together various decisions will be made. In different situations different members will take the lead and the person making the major decisions will vary. As the doctor has the knowledge and skill he will make the clinical decisions. Decisions relating to spiritual support will be made by the spiritual adviser. If the social worker has visited the patient's home she or he will know when it may be suitable for the patient to return. The nurse in charge of the ward must be seen to make the nursing decisions and must never use the team to avoid making these decisions. Some decisions will be joint ones.

So long as all team members are competent at their job, they are in the best position to make the decisions which relate to the specific service that they provide for patient care but the patient must always be involved in these decisions.

Home visits

During rehabilitation following a cerebrovascular accident, amputation or other disabling illness, it is often of value for the patient to return home for a short period prior to discharge. This gives the health care team an opportunity, together with the patient and relatives, to discuss and assess the patient's needs once home.

The visit can be arranged by the registered nurse, physiotherapist, occupational therapist or social worker following discussion at the multidisciplinary team meeting, and after talking to the patient and relatives to explain the purpose of the visit. One or more of the health care workers may accompany the patient, and the community nurse or home help organizer may also be involved. Transport is usually by taxi but will depend on the hospital policy.

Advice may be given to patient and relatives about what to expect once home, and ways of overcoming any problems identified. Arrangement of kitchen, location of toilet and bathroom, height of chairs and bed, and whether the patient can manage any steps or stairs will be examined. Any adjustments or fitments, or extra equipment identified, will then be organized either in liaison with the local authority or community nursing service, or both.

Topics for discussion

1. When a true multidisciplinary ward round takes place, the number of doctors and health care workers taking part can be great. This can be daunting for the patients.

Discuss the role of the nurse in a multidisciplinary ward round. The nurse on the ward round is often held responsible for the preparation of notes, results and X-rays. Discuss how this might affect his or her role in relation to the patients.

2. One of the most common complaints of district nurses relates to the discharge of patients to the care of the community nurses without due notice and with inadequate information, dressings and appliances.

Review the practice of district nurse referral on your ward and discuss ways in which it could be improved to reduce the incidence of these occurrences.

References and Recommended Reading

Autton, N. (1981) *A Handbook of Sick Visiting*. London, Mowbray.

Bennett, G. (1979) *Patients and their Doctors*, Baillière Tindall, London.

Butrym, Z.T. (1976) *The Nature of Social Work*, Macmillan, London.

Clarke, J. & Hiller, R.B. (1975) *Community Care*, H.M. & M. Publishers, Nursing Modules Services, Aylesbury.

Florence Nightingale's *Letter to Mary Jones* (1987) (quoted in Abel-Smith, op-cit., pp. 25 and para. 150 of the Report of the Committee on Nursing – Chairman Asa Briggs HMSO (1972) London.

Friend, P. *Nursing in Primary Health Care*. (DHSS CNO(77)8).

Gee, J.L. & Gee, R.C. (eds) (1983) *Handbook of Community Nursing* Asgard Publishing Company, London.

Keywood, O. (1979) *Nursing in the Community*. Baillière Tindall, London.

Kratz, C. (1978) *Care of the Long Term Sick in the Community*. Churchill Livingstone, London.

Luker, K. & Orr, J. (1985) *Health Visiting* (2nd ed.) Blackwell Scientific Publications, Oxford.

Royal College of Nursing (1988) *Specialities in Nursing – a Report of the working party investigating the development of specialities within the nursing profession*, Royal College of Nursing, London.

Turton, P. & Orr, J. (1985) *Learning to Care in the Community*. Hodder and Stoughton, London.

Chapter 9
Continuing care

Continuing care has become the term used to refer to the care of patients who are dying of their disease, but in the true sense of the words, it means the on-going care of the patient whether this is in the community, in another institution, on return to the outpatient department or in a different part of the hospital. It may also mean the care of the patient and his family to enable maximum quality of life as death approaches, whether this is a long way off, or expected to take only a short time.

This chapter covers continuing care in its broadest sense and so will provide some information about planning for the discharge or transfer of a patient as well as a brief introduction to the topic of 'Care of the dying patient and his family'.

Planning the discharge of a patient

The care and support the patient will require when discharged from hospital must be assessed as early as possible so that the transition from hospital to community is smooth and none of the patient's needs are overlooked. Indeed, preparation for discharge should begin when taking the initial nursing history, ensuring that details of the support available at home and the home environment are assessed. It is essential to refer patients to other health care workers as soon as possible, and this is emphasized in Chapter 8. All those involved in the patient's care need to be made aware of the discharge date as soon as it is known.

Patients feel secure whilst in hospital, partly because help and advice are readily available but also because they are under constant observation by trained personnel. Once back home many patients feel threatened and insecure, and the disruption caused to the patient and the family may be great even if the patient has been in hospital for only a few days. This emphasizes the need for proper and thoughtful planning of the patient's discharge, with provision of adequate and appropriate follow-up support once home.

When planning for the patient's discharge it is the sister or charge nurse or the patient's own nurse who acts as the coordinator (Fig. 9.1), and who finalizes the plans. Nonetheless, this role will be shared with others, depending upon the degree of involvement by other members of the health care team. It must be emphasized that if plans, once made, are altered, and the discharge or transfer cancelled or rearranged, then everyone involved must be made aware of the changes.

Certain steps must be taken when the patient's discharge from hospital is arranged, and these steps are appropriate whether the patient has been in hospital for a short or a long stay. Obviously, the detail of each step will vary depending upon the needs of each patient.

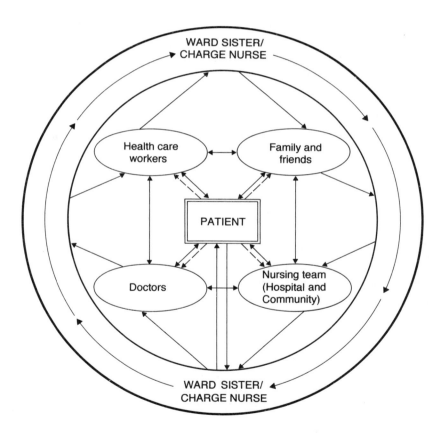

Fig. 9.1 The Complexity of the communication involved when planning discharge from hospital, the ward sister/charge nurse acting as the coordinator.

These steps are:

- Liaising with the patient and the doctor and arranging a suitable date
- Discussing discharge arrangements with the patient
- Liaising with the patient's relatives or friends
- Checking what care is available immediately on return home
- Liaising with other health care workers
- Arranging transport
- Arranging attendance at the outpatient department
- Arranging drugs, dressings, lotions required at home
- Arranging the doctor's letter for the patient's general practitioner
- Obtaining valuables, clothes and suitcase
- Providing medical certificates and completing benefit forms.

All discharges from hospital should be carried out as a planned procedure so that everyone is able to make adequate preparations. Unfortunately, because of the demand for hospital beds, patients are often discharged home at very short notice. Many of these patients are at risk once back in the community as it is often difficult to arrange supporting services at short notice. It is the responsibility of the nurse to ensure that the date set by the doctor is a suitable date, within reason, for the patient, his or her relatives and other health care workers to make appropriate arrangements. If the nurse is forced by the doctor to accept a date which is too early, thereby putting the patient at risk, she or he is not fulfilling the role of the trained nurse. The sister or charge nurse may be in a better position than the more junior nurses, to negotiate for an appropriate discharge date, and should mediate when there is a dispute. Junior doctors must be encouraged to plan ahead when considering the patient's discharge date, bearing in mind admission days and 'emergency take' days. To ensure that the transfer home or to another hospital goes smoothly, one person – sister or charge nurse or the patient's named nurse – should be responsible for checking that all necessary action has been taken well before the patient is ready to leave.

Patient teaching

One fundamental aim of care should be to restore independence to the level attained prior to the patient's present illness. This will not always be possible, but planning care to achieve this should begin as soon as practicable and well before discharge. This will involve teaching patients and often relatives.

Identifying and meeting the learning needs of patients and relatives before discharge has been shown to reduce anxiety, partly because it highlights any worries the patient may have about going home. Wilson-

Barnett and other researchers have shown that this will also reduce anxiety about the effects of treatment and what has been done, and improve the patient's coping ability.

All health care workers who are involved in helping and supporting the patient, must be involved as early as possible in preparing the patient for discharge. This may involve teaching relatives, e.g. the physiotherapist is the best person to teach a relative to lift a patient who has had a cerebrovascular accident. A home visit may also be indicated when teaching a patient and relative to re-adapt once home (see Chapter 8).

Teaching the patient includes imparting knowledge, teaching skills and helping to change attitudes, for example:

Knowledge

- What has been done whilst in hospital
- Effects of treatment
- Drug therapy when at home – reasons for taking and effects of, when to take, where and how to store, special precautions, e.g. steroids, anticoagulants, insulin
- Symptoms to expect once home, e.g. hypoglycaemia if diabetic, excessive tiredness following major surgery
- Level of activity once home.

Skills

- Dressing and undressing
- Feeding
- Walking with or without help
- Climbing stairs
- Kitchen activities
- Giving an injection, e.g. insulin
- Testing urine
- Fitting and coping with an appliance, e.g. stoma bag, breast prosthesis, artificial limb
- Coping with a paralysed limb or limbs
- Coping with haemodialysis.

Attitudes

- Learning to accept and live with a disability, e.g. loss of a limb, blindness
- Complying with treatment, e.g. drugs, special diet
- To stop smoking
- Health education (when relevant).

Adequate, easily assimilated information, giving the reasons for a course of treatment or action, will help the patient to modify attitudes and become more positive. It often helps the patient and his family if this information is written down. Leaflets and booklets are available from the Health Education Council, British Heart Foundation, etc. which are of value and can be used for reference once home. Information leaflets produced by ward staff for a specific group of patients are also useful.

Discussion with the patient and doctor

It is not sufficient to assume that, because the doctor has discussed the patient's discharge at the bedside, the patient is aware of the proposed discharge date. It is necessary for the nurse to have further discussion with the patient in order to decide a definite date. If not, it may be found that a patient who is to be discharged in two days' time has already telephoned a relative and arranged transport home for that day. On the other hand, it might be discovered that it would be of less risk to the patient if discharge is delayed for a few days. Confusion can easily arise as the patient is often excited by the thought of going home. If adequate assessment has been made of the patient's home conditions – the help available, location of the toilet, location of the bedroom, etc. – on and during admission, any needs arising from inadequate help or facilities available will already have been planned for. This will include such things as home help, commode, meals-on-wheels, etc. It is, however essential to involve the patient in these decisions.

Liaising with relatives

Relatives or friends who will be concerned with last minute arrangements, such as providing transport or perishable foodstuffs and warming the house if the patient lives alone, need to have the date of discharge confirmed as quickly as possible. This must be confirmed by the person in charge of the ward or the nurse responsible for the patient's care, and not left to the patient. If the nursing team is not involved the discharge will not be coordinated and certain aspects may be overlooked.

It will be necessary for the relatives to be aware of the extent or limits of the activity which can be undertaken by the patient. For example, if a man has had a myocardial infarction his wife will need to know over what period of time and in which ways his activity is to be increased.

The nurse has a responsibility to make clear to relatives what to expect once the patient is at home. It is very important that they should be aware of the rate of progress to be expected, the degree of discomfort or pain the patient may experience, possible problems or setbacks which may occur and when to be concerned and send for the general practitioner.

Relatives will also need to know how to cope with stomas, special appliances, application of lotions and administration of drugs, both oral and injections, especially in the case of children, the mentally subnormal and vague, elderly patients.

Liaising with other health care workers

In an efficiently managed ward all health care workers who are able to provide help and support for the patient will have had contact with the patient and possibly the family during the patient's stay in hospital. Each one must be notified of the proposed date of discharge once known.

The patient may need to attend the physiotherapy department, speech therapy or occupational therapy department following discharge home and liaison with physiotherapist, speech therapist or occupational therapist is necessary in order to arrange an appointment. An ambulance may be required and this must also be arranged. The physiotherapist may have provided the patient with various aids, such as walking frame or crutches, and the patient must know whether these are to be taken home and where to return them when they are no longer needed.

If the patient has been having a special diet the dietician will have explained this in detail to the patient and possibly to his or her relatives, but the dietician may need to see the patient again before discharge home.

Liaison with the community nursing service as described in Chapter 8 will be finalized once the discharge date has been arranged and a referral letter, in the case of the district nurse, is completed and given to the patient or relatives to pass on to the district nurse. Some health authorities may prefer district nurse letters to be posted. In the case of dressings to wounds, a small supply of dressings and the appropriate lotion must be supplied.

Plans made for home help, meals-on-wheels, etc., need to be finalized once the discharge date is known. If the patient is dependent on social services it is often better to discharge the patient after, rather than at the weekend. If convalescence has been agreed upon, the date of transfer to the convalescent home will determine the discharge date. The necessary transport will need to be arranged.

Any patient who is fitted with an appliance should be confident about the care of the appliance before going home. This includes information about where and how to obtain the necessary equipment (such as stoma bags) or replacement appliances (such as breast prostheses) should the need arise. There are other appliances which may be required, such as callipers, surgical footwear, artificial limbs, spinal supports, artificial eyes, ears and noses, elastic hosiery, wigs and wheelchairs. All special appliances require a consultant's signed requisition, and in some cases a special form is required. Appliances required for home nursing, such as commodes, backrests and special mattresses, are usually supplied on loan by the health authority. Arrangements for these are made by the social worker or, following discharge, the district nurse.

If a patient is chronically or terminally ill and his or her relatives want to nurse the patient at home, it may be felt that a night nursing service will be of help and support to the family. This service can be arranged through the community nursing service, local voluntary groups, the local authority or the Marie Curie Memorial Foundation (see Appendix II). The social worker or liaison district nurse will be able to provide advice on this. The British Red Cross Society and the St John Ambulance Brigade are also able to loan articles.

Transport

Appropriate transport arrangements must be made. In some cases an ambulance may be indicated, especially if the patient is bedridden or has impaired mobility and has several steps to negotiate. In some areas at least 48 hours' notice is requested whenever possible by the ambulance service, and this enhances the need for proper planned discharges. If the patient is to go home by ambulance the nurse must ensure that someone will be at home to receive the patient or, alternatively, that the patient has a doorkey.

Many relatives are able to arrange their own transport if this is discussed with them. It may need to be stressed that it is not essential that the patient leaves the ward at 10.00 hours and a time suitable to the relative or friend can be negotiated. In some hospitals a car service may be available.

Appointments

Some hospitals arrange follow-up appointments before the patient leaves so that the appointment card can be given to the patient and the arrangements explained. Other hospitals inform patients of their appointments by post. Another important consideration when planning discharge is to ascertain that the patient is able to get to the outpatient department. Many patients are able to provide their own transport or travel by bus or train. Others, who are less fit, or live in a country district without a regular bus, will require transport such as car service or ambulance and will need to know what time to be ready.

Some patients may have more than one appointment if they have been treated by more than one specialist, or they may also have an appointment to see one of the specialist nurses.

Prescriptions and dressings

It is an advantage to the pharmacy department if the patient's discharge prescription is made available to them before the day of discharge. Many hospitals have a restriction on the number of tablets they are able to supply to a patient. The limit may be a fortnight's supply. Nevertheless, in certain circumstances, for example, a patient who is housebound and lives alone, this may be extended if an explanation is given to the pharmacist.

Dressings and lotions which may be required are usually obtained on the prescription. It is important that the patient takes adequate dressings to allow time for the district nurse to obtain a prescription from the patient's general practitioner for a further supply.

It is essential that the patient, or relatives, or both, understand the drug therapy and regimes before leaving the ward. In some cases it may be necessary for the nurse to write this out for them.

The patient will need to be aware of any special instructions relating to the drug therapy as with insulin, steroids, monoamine oxidase inhibitors and anticoagulants and be provided with the appropriate card to carry. In these situations it is to the patient's advantage to be instructed about the drugs and the importance of carrying the card during his or her stay in hospital and not on the day of discharge. This should apply to all drug therapy. The patient will need to know how long the supply of drugs will last and how to obtain subsequent supplies.

General practitioner's letter

The letter to the patient's general practitioner is either written by the doctor before the patient leaves the ward and given to the patient or relatives, or it is written after discharge and posted. If given to the relatives or patient it should ensure that the general practitioner is immediately alerted in case of an emergency arising once the patient is at home as he or she will have the necessary information available to him or her.

Ward clerks or ward secretaries usually order ambulances, make appointments and ensure that the doctor's letter is made available for the house officer or registrar to complete. Nevertheless, it is the ultimate responsibility of the sister or charge nurse to see that these tasks are completed, so it is necessary for the nurse to inform the ward clerk of all known discharge dates and the appointments and ambulances required as early as possible. In the absence of a ward clerk, this often becomes the responsibility of the nurse in charge.

Obtaining valuables, clothes and suitcase

If valuables such as cash, jewellery, pension books or bank books have been taken for safe-keeping, these must be obtained prior to discharge. It is important to think ahead, for if the patient is going home in the evening or at the weekend, it may not be possible for the valuables to be retrieved from the hospital safe. The procedure for obtaining such items will vary from hospital to hospital but, in most instances, will include obtaining a signature from the patient once the valuables have been returned.

In the more modern hospitals the patient's clothes and suitcase may be stored in a wardrobe near the patient's bed area. In other hospitals clothing and suitcases may be stored either centrally and returned to the patient by a designated person, or stored in a ward annexe. In all situations the nurse must ensure that these are returned to the patient, and the necessary forms signed if required.

Medical certificates and benefit forms

A sickness benefit claim form is completed by the patient for the first week of sickness, a sick note not being required from the doctor or hospital until after the seventh day. To claim, the patient must have been sick for at least four consecutive days, including Sunday, if claiming statutory Sick Pay, but excluding Sunday if claiming Sickness Benefit.

Nursing staff are able to complete and sign the yellow National Insurance Hospital Inpatient Certificates, necessary after the first week of sickness, which should also be given to the patient on the day of discharge as well as during the patient's stay in hospital. The patient or relatives must be instructed to obtain another medical certificate from the general practitioner within the next week. When a patient attends as an outpatient the National Insurance Certificate, which is white, must be signed by a doctor.

Some patients will ask for a private medical certificate. The format of these vary from hospital to hospital and can usually be completed by a trained nurse.

Some patients belong to private insurance or benefit schemes and obtain claim forms from the appropriate office or their employer. The forms usually state clearly whether a doctor's or trained nurse's signature is required. Most forms also require the official hospital stamp.

In long-stay hospitals staff may be asked by relatives to sign or witness their signatures on certain documents such as life insurance policies in the event of the death of either the patient or the patient's spouse. These situations are usually referred to the hospital administrator.

Once the patient has left the hospital the nursing records are completed in detail, including the general condition of the patient, time of discharge, mode of transport, whether the patient was accompanied, instructions given to the patient and relatives, outpatient appointments and any special arrangements which have been made, for example, if a referral has been made to the district nurse. Some structured nursing reports will include a section relating to the patient's discharge from hospital.

Case notes, including those of other hospitals, are returned to the medical records department and the X-rays to the X-ray department. The ward clerk or secretary usually attends to this, but if there is no ward clerk they are sent in a sealed envelope to the appropriate department via the messenger service.

If the patient is a private patient, the private patient's clerk or secretary is informed. In the case of a serviceman or woman the appropriate authority is notified via the medical records officer or hospital administrator, and the patient is usually instructed to return to his or her base, unit or ship.

Any drugs or lotions that have been dispensed for an individual patient whilst an inpatient are returned to the pharmacy. Special diets are cancelled. Any special equipment loaned to the patient by the physiotherapist or occupational therapist which is not required by the patient at home, is returned to the appropriate department.

Transfer of a patient

When patients are to transfer to another ward or another hospital the news of the proposed move often causes the patient acute anxiety. It is essential, therefore, that careful thought is given to the way the news is given, and by whom. The nurse in charge of the ward is usually the best person to do this. In many hospitals 'sleeping out' of patients from one ward to another is practised in order to create empty beds, and this is accepted as the norm by many nurses who perhaps give little thought to the distressing effect it has on both patients and their relatives.

When transferring patients, good communication between all persons concerned with the transfer is of vital importance.

Within the hospital

When a patient is transferred from one ward to another the following steps are taken:

- Discuss with the patient
- Notify the relatives
- Contact the receiving ward
- Assess whether the patient is to walk, go by chair, or in the bed
- Notify the portering service
- Ensure nursing records are completed and up-to-date
- Help the patient to pack together personal belongings
- Assess whether it is necessary for a nurse to accompany the patient
- Inform the admissions office
- Inform the switchboard if they keep a list of inpatients
- Ensure that the nursing report, medical notes, X-rays, drugs specifically dispensed for the patient, diet sheet and observation charts are placed in an envelope and sent with the patient, together with the patient's personal belongings.

To another hospital

When a patient is transferred to another hospital the following steps are taken:

- Discuss with the patient
- Notify the relatives of the intention to transfer, the hospital, its location and the ward
- Contact the receiving ward
- Arrange transport
- Assess whether a nurse escort is required and, if so, ensure that the nurse is able to get back as it cannot be assumed that the ambulance will be returning or will be able to accommodate the nurse
- Write a nursing transfer letter
- Ensure that the doctor writes a medical transfer letter with all relevant medical information
- Help the patient to pack together all personal belongings
- Obtain any valuables held by the hospital for safe-keeping
- Complete any benefit forms the patient may require
- Inform the admissions office
- Inform the switchboard if indicated.

In some hospitals it is the procedure to send medical notes and X-rays. If so, the medical records department and the X-ray department must be notified that these have been sent out of the hospital. Some hospitals send a copy of the medical notes.

Discharge against medical advice

If the nurse takes the time to sit and listen it is often discovered that patients who want to discharge themselves are often distressed by some particular incident or situation. For example, some people find it difficult to sleep in a room with others, or they feel they are not able to obtain the information they need, or are worried about their family at home. Therefore they react by wanting to leave, and take their own discharge.

Often it is possible to solve the problems so that the patient then feels able to stay and continue treatment. In some instances it may be necessary to call on the assistance of a close relative or friend of the patient who may be able to persuade the patient to stay. If the patient is determined to leave the hospital the doctor is notified. The doctor may be able to reason with the patient and persuade the patient to continue treatment. If this is not possible, it is the doctor's responsibility to explain to the patient that the hospital will take no further responsibility and obtain a signed statement from the patient on a special form.

When patients discharge themselves from hospital, the hospital has no legal obligation to continue treatment or provide a follow-up service. Nevertheless, each situation is assessed on its own merits.

Care of the dying patient and the family

Dying remains one of the few certainties in life today

(Marks, 1988)

Attitudes to death and to the dying have changed dramatically over the years. Until this century, death was expected and accepted, and was often a public event, taking place in the company of family and friends. During this century, partly due to the advances of medical technology and improvements in nutrition and public health, death has come to be viewed as the failure of life. It has become a forbidden subject for conversation (Gorer, 1967) with the result that many people now feel unable to cope with the basic care of the dying person at home. By 1984, 68 per cent of all deaths in the United Kingdom took place in hospital (Office of Population Censuses and Statistics, 1984).

Hospital deaths are often impersonal and technology-orientated, but people at home may be isolated and have inadequate symptom control

(Marks, 1988). This has resulted in the development of the hospice movement through the 1970s and 1980s, to combine the best of home and hospital care. Most recently, there has been the development of teams of home care nurses who offer skilled nursing, expert advice on symptom control and emotional support to patients and their families at home. There have also developed hospital support teams of nurses who provide expert advice on symptom control and support while the patient is in hospital, and sometimes these nurses continue their support when the patient is discharged to the community.

The ward sister or charge nurse needs to consider how best to help several different groups through death and bereavement. The first priority is the patient. The family or relatives also need practical and emotional support both prior to and after the death has taken place. The nursing team and other health professionals will also need practical and emotional support, as this is a stressful time. Lastly, the ward sister herself, or the charge nurse, needs to be sure that she or he gets support from whatever sources possible (Fig. 9.2).

The patient

People are frightened of death, or more accurately people are afraid of what the 'dying' might entail. Most dying patients (Davidson, 1979) express concern about:

(1)   Fear that the family will be abandoned
(2)   Loss of self-management and independence
(3)   Fear of pain and other intractable symptoms

People will cope with impending death in exactly the same way that they cope with other crises in their lives, but their ability to cope will also depend on how well their symptoms can be alleviated.

Many terminally ill patients are afraid of pain, nausea, vomiting, dyspnoea, incontinence and insomnia. There are now many techniques available to the nurse to alleviate these miserable symptoms with the help and cooperation of the doctor. Pain, for example, must be anticipated and analgesia given in adequate doses at regular intervals *before* the pain comes on, in order to keep the patient pain-free. The dying patient may be unable or feel unwilling to complain of pain even though pain exists. The nurse must be particularly sensitive to these patients and ensure that adequate analgesia is given at all times. The type, dose and frequency of the analgesia must be discussed at frequent intervals with the patient and doctor concerned.

Communication with a dying person can be difficult as the nurse may

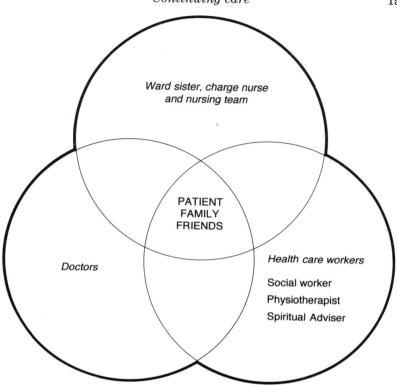

Fig. 9.2 The communication and support network for the dying patient and family and friends.

be unsure what level of acceptance of death has been reached by the patient. At first, people are often totally unaware that they are dying. At this stage it is possible for staff and relatives to collude in keeping it from them but this is rarely a successful ploy for long. Gradually, the patient becomes suspicious as the gravity of his condition becomes more apparent, but at this stage he still does not usually ask questions nor seek confirmation. Later still, there is often a period of mutual pretence where the patient has realized that he is dying and the staff and family feel that he has 'guessed' but the situation is not yet discussed openly. The stage of open awareness of impending death, where the patient, staff and relatives openly admit their knowledge allows more free discussion and sharing of feelings. The patient often feels that he once again has control over his life (Glaser and Strauss, 1964). The stage of awareness of impending death has a great effect on the ability of the nurses to talk with the patient about his feelings, behaviour and anxieties, and requires well-developed assessment and communication skills. In making their assessment of the patient the nurses may be helped by an understanding of the stages through which a person passes on the way to acceptance of death. Elizabeth Kubler-Ross (1969) described these stages and has also highlighted many of the emotions and anxieties faced by the dying individual. The stages of dying are not seen as a continuum; a person may go through one stage and then return to it again later, or omit stages altogether; another person may experience several stages at the same time. Elizabeth Kubler-Ross draws attention to the following stages:

(1) **Denial**
   - Existential denial: the belief that mortality is not threatened.
   - Psychological denial: 'It's not true' – exemplified by the patient who just forgets that he has been told and continually seeks reassurance.
   - Non-attention denial: the person who has accepted impending death, but prefers to pretend that it is not going to happen. It makes living less painful, without having to continuously think about death.
(2) **Anger**
(3) **Bargaining**
(4) **Depression:**   it may be difficult to distinguish 'normal' depression, that is an appropriate reaction, from a clinical or treatable depression.
(5) **Anticipatory grief:**   as a result of achieving a high level of symptom control, the dying person may be free to contemplate what he is losing (Stedeford, 1985).
(6) **Acceptance:**   a stage of peaceful acceptance may be the ultimate aim for some patients. However, in many cases acceptance is more often exemplified by a sort of resignation and desire for escape from the weariness and exhaustion. The person's personality, age, religious belief and the degree of support s/he receives from family and friends all help to determine how easily impending death can be accepted.
(7) **Hope:**   as has been previously described (non-attention denial) it is possible to hold two incompatible ideas at the same time. This means that the argument for withholding the truth from patients, that it will destroy hope, is unfounded, as those who do not want to hear the truth will deny it. However, without hope, life is meaningless, so the dying person should be encouraged to hope for attainable targets.

Mental anguish is a very real problem for the dying. Patients can be frightened of dying alone, upset by the grief of their relatives and friends, worried about lack or loss of religious conviction, and worried about sorting out their business affairs, financial problems and providing for their families. The nurse must be able to anticipate these fears and anxieties which can be reduced by allowing the patients to talk and express their worries. This means that the nurse in charge must show the patients that she or he has time to sit and listen, and must encourage the other members of the team to do the same. Nurses often worry that if they put themselves in such a situation they will be unable to answer questions that the patient may ask, but in many instances the patient will not expect answers. The patient's main need is to talk and be listened to. For the nurse just to be there with the patient is often enough.

Some patients will show signs of severe loss – the impending loss of life – and this may lead to defective communication. The nurse must observe closely for signs that the patient wants to unburden himself or herself. One obvious sign is that the patient becomes withdrawn or weepy. Other signs are less obvious. In these situations the nurse must encourage the patient to express these fears and anxieties.

The nursing team can be a source of valuable support by treating dying patients as normal human beings and involving them in decision-making related to their care. A simple example is whether the patient wants to sit out of bed, get dressed, or have a bath.

The nurse's approach must be one of care and respect. This is conveyed by spending time with the patient and talking about everyday events and inviting the patient's opinions. Physical contact will convey to the patient that the nurse cares.

If the patient is feeling angry or hostile this may be directed at the nursing team. Anger or hostility must always be met with calmness and understanding – never with anger. The patient's aggression may be directed at the family who will need reassurance that, although distressing, this is a normal reaction and is not a personal attack on them. It occurs because the patient is frightened and needs family and friends at hand.

Moving the dying patient into a single room may increase the patient's distress; it should never be allowed to become ward policy and must not be carried out indiscriminately. Some patients prefer the privacy of a single room, especially if the family is present. Other patients who are distressed physically may increase the anxiety of the other patients in the ward. Nevertheless, the wishes of the dying patient should always be respected and contact with other patients is extremely important. The patient should be encouraged to maintain existing social contact so that he or she does not feel cast out. This will involve allowing friends to visit at reasonable times, even if outside hospital visiting times.

Persisting with unnecessary procedures such as recording temperature and blood pressure may cause further distress to a dying patient who is perhaps confused or semi-conscious and should be discouraged if serving no useful purpose. On the other hand, it may sometimes be important to continue with such procedures if the patient benefits psychologically.

It is important that other members of the caring team are involved in this stage of the patient's life. The social worker can give practical assistance and support to the patient who is worrying about the financial implications of death. The social worker, as counsellor, is also able to support the patient through the various emotions associated with dying. Other patients may obtain support and comfort from the hospital spiritual adviser. Early referral is essential and it is often the ward sister or charge nurse who must suggest that other health care workers are involved.

It is important to practising Roman Catholics that they receive from the priest Anointment of the Sick when seriously ill, and for many Protestants Holy Communion is very meaningful. An Orthodox Jew must have either the rabbi or family members present when dying, and after death non-Jews are not allowed to touch the body. Priests, nuns and monks are usually supported by their fellow priests or nuns at the time of death, who will, after death, dress the person in their vestments.

Moslems are supported, when dying, by their families, and Buddhists by a priest. Immediately following death, the Moslem's head is raised on a pillow and turned to face Mecca, the body being touched only by those of the Moslem faith. Likewise Hindus and Sikhs are only touched by other Hindus and Sikhs.

In the United Kingdom, there are now more people who hold religious and cultural beliefs which are different from the traditional ones. It is important that these are identified as soon as possible after admission, so that the patient's beliefs can be adhered to.

The family

As soon as it becomes obvious that the patient is in the terminal stages of the illness, with the patient's permission, the family should be made aware of this. It may be necessary to arrange interviews with the doctor, but this will need to be followed-up by the nurse. The nurse may need to spend a lot of time with them, explaining gently and carefully, leaving no possibility for misinterpretation, and answering their many questions and allaying their fears. It will be necessary to repeat what has been said, possibly using different ways to explain the same thing. Tact and patience will be needed as, the first time of hearing, the family will probably be unable to assimilate all the relevant facts. Their communication may be impaired because of the impending loss.

Relatives and friends are often distressed by physical and psychological changes in the patient, making it most important that they are encouraged to talk about the patient when in good health. It is very difficult to help a relative come to terms with marked physical changes which may occur, for example, when a patient has been taking large doses of steroids.

In the very end stages, just prior to death occurring, changes in the patient's condition which are obvious to the nurse may be less apparent to the lay person and not necessarily recognized with the same gravity, so all changes in the patient's condition must be explained to the family. The family should always be given the opportunity to stay at the bedside so that they are present at the time of death, consequently they must be informed immediately of any sudden change in condition. This can be done either by telephone, telephone message via a neighbour or friend or, as a last resort, by police message. The police usually ask the relatives to contact the hospital immediately. It is wise to suggest that someone accompanies the nearest relatives when they come to the hospital. In the event of sudden or unexpected death relatives should be sent for and never told over the telephone.

Decisions made between the patient's relatives and nurses must be communicated to all nurses. In some instances relatives ask that, in the event of death occurring during the night, they are not contacted until the morning. Wishes like this must be respected and conveyed to the night nursing team, and also recorded in the nursing report.

Relatives, too, need to feel cared for and, again, communication by touch can be very comforting. Relatives and friends must feel able to cry without embarrassment. They may have fears and anxieties about the actual process of dying, wondering what it will be like. Their fears may be influenced by the media or by past experiences. The nurse can help by listening and reassuring them, and being open and honest. The relatives can also be helped by being encouraged to be themselves.

At this time the family will also worry about the practicalities associated with a death in the family. It has been shown that advice given to relatives before death helps to avoid adverse reactions during the bereavement period.

Other health care workers should be involved in the support of the family, especially as they are often able to visit the family at home following the death. Early referral is vital.

Some relatives may feel guilt or anger which may be directed at the hospital, the nurses, the doctors or other health care workers. They may need to talk through this guilt or voice their anger, which will help them to come to terms with themselves and their bereavement. Their anger must never be taken personally.

Relatives can be helped to overcome the feeling of helplessness if given the opportunity to take part in decision-making and in the patient's care. Relatives can be encouraged to help the patient at mealtimes or, if the patient is unable to eat or drink, they can be shown how to keep the patient's lips moist. This will also enhance communication between patient and relatives and provide a source of support. If relatives are sitting at the bedside, cotsides, although sometimes a necessity, will create a barrier and should be removed as long as they are replaced when the patient is alone.

The closest relatives appreciate being able to stay close at hand, especially as death approaches. It is becoming more common for hospitals to provide accommodation for this purpose but if this facility is not available the offer of an easy chair in the dayroom is usually acceptable. Some relatives prefer to stay at the bedside.

If staying over a long period the relatives become very tired and often irritable. Irritability and awkwardness must be met with kindness, tact and understanding. The patient may also be irritable, especially if frightened or in pain, and this may cause further distress and misunderstanding for the family. They will need to talk this through with the sister or charge nurse who must help them to understand that this is an expected reaction.

At the time of death, bereavement will be demonstrated in a variety of ways. All relatives will be stunned and shocked whether death is unexpected or otherwise. They may faint, or become agitated and scream and shout. Others may become angry and unable to make rational decisions. Others outwardly appear cool and able to make rational judgements. This should never be mistaken for lack of concern – it is usually a sign of delayed shock. If a nurse is present to listen to and comfort the relatives, this is often very supportive. A cup of tea or coffee will also help.

Most bereaved relatives need to be given the opportunity to return to the bedside to convince themselves that the patient has died and, in many cases, they appreciate being left alone for a while. In the case of babies and children it is not unusual for the parents to pick the child up and hold it close to them. This helps them to realize that the child has died. The relatives should never be rushed away from the hospital but allowed to leave in their own time, as they often feel the need to stay a while to gather their thoughts and come to terms with things. When a patient dies in a ward or room with other patients it is important that the other patients are told as soon as possible that death has occurred.

At the time of death practical help is sought by the relatives and will include the following:

- Registration of the death
- Contacting the undertaker
- Collection of personal effects.

Registration of death

In England all deaths must be registered within five days at the office of the Registrar of Births, Deaths and Marriages in the district where the death has occurred. The office is usually open from 9.00 a.m. to 4.30 p.m., Monday to Friday, although special arrangements may be made for registration on Saturday mornings. The registration is made by taking the medical certificate which has been completed by the certifying doctor and issued by the hospital to the registrar's office. Whoever is to register the death should be advised to also take the birth and marriage certificates, pension book – if applicable – and National Insurance card of the deceased, as certain information in these documents will be required. The registrar then issues a death certificate authorizing the undertaker to remove the body from the hospital, a form to enable relatives to claim for a death grant through the Department of Social Security and, if necessary, forms to enable insurance policies to be claimed.

Contacting the undertaker

Relatives should be advised to contact the undertaker as soon as possible as in most cases the undertaker will then make all the necessary arrangements and advise the relatives. If the relatives state that they are either unwilling, or cannot afford to pay for the funeral, or if relatives cannot be traced, the hospital administrator should be notified straight away. In certain circumstances the hospital authorities can arrange and pay for the funeral, and the administrator must register the death.

In the case of cremation, special forms are required and the undertaker will attend to this. Two doctors' certificates certifying the cause of death must be at the crematorium 24 hours before the cremation can take place, so that they can be examined by the crematorium's medical referee.

Collection of personal effects

If the relatives ask for any jewellery to be left on the body this is usually written on the identification label attached to the body, and is also listed with the other property. Some hospitals require a form of indemnity to be signed by the next of kin.

All personal effects, including any valuables, are listed in the appropriate property book and then either taken to the administrator's department and given to the relatives or, in some hospitals, handed over to the relatives by the ward sister or charge nurse or deputy. Care must always be taken as personal effects must be handed to the legal next of kin who must sign the property book. If there is any doubt at all about the next of kin the administrator must be contacted. Advice, if required, is readily available from the district or regional solicitor.

Although the social worker can put bereaved relatives in contact with voluntary organizations it is an advantage that the person in charge of the ward is also aware of organizations available locally, such as Cruse, National Association of Widows or the Compassionate Friends (see Appendix II).

Care of the family and relatives of the deceased does not end when they leave the hospital. They should always be given a telephone number of someone to contact for further information should they require it, and many places now offer some sort of bereavement counselling or back-up.

Adaptation to the loss of a loved one is a normal and essential process. Grief can be both physically and emotionally traumatic, but it plays an essential part in the return to a normal and healthy lifestyle. Worden (1983) describes the tasks of mourning as:

(1) to accept the reality of the loss
(2) to experience the pain of grief
(3) to adjust to an environment in which the deceased is missing
(4) to withdraw emotional energy and reinvest it in another relationship.

These must all be accomplished before adjustment to bereavement is complete. An understanding of the importance of the expression of pain, loss and grief can help nurses to be compassionate when dealing with the bereaved. Perhaps it is a pity that mourning rituals have changed as they had great benefits in offering an acceptable place for the release of emotions and saying goodbye.

The ward team

Sensitivity on the part of the sister or charge nurse will show her or his awareness of the need of the nursing team for support during terminal illness and death, and a willingness to provide this. Much distress is caused by the conflict between curing and caring which can result in some nurses feeling that death is a failure. It must be stressed that this is not usually so, but is a normal part of life. Senior nurses should be sympathetic to the anxiety shown, not only by student nurses, but also by the trained nurses and auxiliary nurses in the team.

To help staff through this anxious, distressing time good communication is vital. The handover can be used to discuss the nurses' anxieties as well as the patient's physical and psychological needs and any signs of anxiety observed by the nurses. If the nurses' fears and worries are discussed by all members of the team and, if possible, other health care workers, the burden will be shared and therefore becomes easier to cope with. It is important that trained nurses as well as students and support nurses discuss their feelings so that everyone is helped. Everyone must be fully aware of the reasons for a certain line of treatment, or changing or stopping treatment. If active treatment is still being given this may be to relieve symptoms and this will need to be explained. A terminally ill patient who is grossly anaemic, for example, may be kept more comfortable if given a blood transfusion. The nursing policy for the patient must also be made clear. If analgesia is prescribed 'as required' but is being given at regular intervals, or if the patient, although obviously dying, is more comfortable in an easy chair, this must be conveyed to the nursing team.

All nurses, especially the less experienced, need to be aware of what might happen at the time of death and how to cope with the situation. For example, if a patient with carcinoma of the lungs is having frequent haemoptyses, the patient may eventually have a massive haemorrhage resulting in death and the nurses need to be aware of the possibility and of what to do if it happens.

It is important that the nurses know that they should listen carefully to the patient and if an answer is needed to try to answer the question truthfully but gently or, if this is not possible, to report to a more senior nurse immediately. Nurses often need to be told that the relatives will also need someone to listen to them and will want an opportunity to talk about the patient, both before and after death has occurred.

Many junior nurses have never seen a dead body and are very afraid at their first encounter with death. First impressions are extremely important and if allowed to assist an understanding, experienced nurse with last offices this will help the nurse come to terms with death. This can be arranged by the sensitive sister or charge nurse. It will also help the nurse if she is encouraged to touch the body.

The ward sister or charge nurse should never be afraid to show concern for the patient, his or her relatives, and staff in this very stressful situation, and always be willing to talk about her or his own fears and anxieties. If a nurse is unable to cope with the situation, she may become cold and abrupt – this will reflect on the patient, the family and on the rest of the nursing team, and the ward sister or charge nurse has the influence to prevent this.

Stress

> Stress is now recognized as a hazard for those employed in the helping and caring professions. At some time or another we can expect to experience emotional and physical problems arising out of the demands of caring for people
>
> (Bailey, 1985)

Within nursing there are many possible causes of stress, which manifests itself in several ways, and adverse mechanisms may be adopted to enable the nurse to cope with the work (see Fig. 9.3).

If exposed to excessive stress, 'burn-out' may occur (Maslach, 1976). Burn-out is a disease of over-commitment, with withdrawal from work in response to dissatisfaction or excessive stress. The health care worker who begins with enthusiasm and high ideals, becomes apathetic. Burn-out can result in fatigue, apathy, absenteeism, and a negative attitude to the job with resistance to contact with patients and colleagues. It is important, therefore, wherever possible, to alleviate stress at work.

Alleviating stress at work

A compassionate ward sister or charge nurse will be sensitive to signs of stress in members of the nursing team and endeavour to alleviate this by:

- Ensuring good lines of communication (see Chapter 2)
- Ensuring nurses have adequate information about patients
- Allowing nurses to express their feelings and fears
- Allowing nurses to talk to their colleagues
- Identifying training needs
- Planning a good induction to the ward for new nurses
- Using counselling facilities if available, e.g. occupational health department, trained counsellor

Causes of Stress in Nursing	Manifestations
Exposure to human suffering	Fatigue
seriously ill young adults	Headaches
sick children and babies	Muscle tension
dying patients	Gastric and bowel problems
confused, aggressive patients	Hypertension
patients in pain	Reduced job satisfaction
mutilated patients – accidents	Role conflict
mutilated patients – surgery	Accident proneness
self-inflicted illness	Anorexia
cancer patients	Overeating
renal patients	Smoking
accident victims	Drinking
stillbirths	Drug-taking
bereaved relatives	Anger
Closer nurse-patient relationships	Anxiety
Helplessness	Depression
Curing v. caring	
Feeling of incompetence	
Lack of support systems	Coping Mechanisms
Lack of resources	Dehumanising the patients
Worker v. learner (students)	Indifference
Manager v. clinician v. teacher (sisters)	Inappropriate laughter
High, often unrealistic, expectations	Denial
High technology equipment	Task allocation
Communication breakdown	Ritualistic and rigid approach
Constant change	Obsession with procedures and rules
Heavy workload (patient care hours	Resistance to change
greater than nursing hours available)	Absenteeism
Uncertainty of how to handle patient's	
questions	

Fig. 9.3 Stress in Nursing.

- Ensuring an even distribution of workload
- Planning duty rotas fairly.

By supporting the nursing team at all times, the ward sister or charge nurse will enable the team members to cope with stress in a positive, rather than a negative way.

On a more personal level, ward sisters and charge nurses may benefit from encouraging their staff, and from adopting for themselves, Vachon's (1978) tips for improving coping skills for staff working with the dying:

(1) Encouragement of personal insight to understand and acknowledge one's own limits
(2) Healthy balance between work and outside life
(3) The promotion of a team approach to care
(4) An ongoing support system within work and outside work
(5) For those working in isolation, continuing guidance and support from peers and superiors.

Topics for discussion

1. Discharge planning

Make a list of the equipment that might be needed by a patient being discharged with a new colostomy.

You are arranging a district nurse to visit this patient at home. Using the forms available at your hospital, write a sample district nurse referral letter, including information about the level of patient education attained and the psychological support that might be needed.

Is there any other information the patient should receive?

2. Care of the dying – care of the relatives

> Rachel was 19 years old and dying from a cerebral tumour. Her father and mother stayed at her bedside during the day and her father also stayed throughout the night. One morning, her mother was extremely angry and critical of the nursing staff on the ward.

Discuss some possible reasons for this anger and how nursing staff might help Rachel's mother to work through it.

3. Staff support

> It was Student Nurse Jones' second day on an adult ward – her first adult nursing experience – when a very sick elderly man died, not unexpectedly. Nurse Jones became very distressed. The sister took her into the office where she began to cry uncontrollably.

If you were the sister in this situation, how would you tackle it? Suggest some possible reasons why this nurse might be so upset. What practical and emotional support would you be able to offer Nurse Jones.

References

Bailey, R.D. (1985) *Coping with Stress in Caring.* Blackwell Scientific Publications, Oxford.

Davidson, G. (1979) 'Hospice care for the dying' in H. Wass (ed.) *Dying, Facing Facts.* McGraw Hill, New York.

Glaser, B. and Strauss, A. (1966) *Awareness of Dying.* Aldine, Chicago.

Gorer, G. (1976) *Death, Grief and Mourning.* Anchor Books, Doubleday and Co., New York.

Kubler-Ross, E. (1969) *On Death and Dying.* Macmillan, New York.

Marks, M. (1988) 'Death, Dying Bereavement and Loss' in Tiffany, R. (series ed.), Webb, P. (ed.) *Oncology for Nurses and Health Care Professionals,* (2nd ed) Vol 2. Harper and Row, London.

Maslach, C. (1976) 'Burned-out' *Human Behaviour*, **5**, 16–22

Office of Population Censuses and Statistics (1984) *Theories*, DH1, Table 14, HMSO, London.

Stedeford, A. (1985) *Facing Death*. Heinemann, London.

Vachon, M. (1978) Motivation and stress experienced by staff working with the terminally ill, *Death Education*. **12**, 113–22.

Worden, J.W. (1983) *Grief Counselling and Grief Therapy*, Tavistock Publications, London.

Recommended Reading

Ainsworth-Smith, I. & Speek, P. (1982) *Caring for the Dying and the Bereaved*. Society for Promoting Christian Knowledge, London.

Charles-Edwards, A. (1983) *The Nursing Care of the Dying Patient*. Beaconsfield Publishers Ltd, Beaconsfield.

Cherniss, C. (1980) *Staff Burn-out: Job Stress in the Human Services*. Sage, London.

Gay, P & Pitkeathley, J. (1979) *When I Went Home – A Study of Patients Discharge from Hospital*. King Edward's Hospital Fund, London.

Gee, J.L. & Gee, R.C. (eds) (1983) *Handbook of Community Nursing* 1983. Asgard Publishing Company, London.

Hockey, L. (1968) *Care in the Balance*. Queen's Institute of District Nursing, London.

McGilloway, O. & Myco, F. (1985) *Nursing and Spiritual Care*. Harper and Row, London.

Murray, Parkes, C. (1972) *Bereavement: Studies of Grief in Adult Life*. Penguin, Harmondsworth.

Neuberger, J. (1987) *Caring for Dying People of Different Faith* Austen Cornish in Association with the Lisa Sainsbury Foundation, London.

Pincus, L. (1981) *Death and the Family*. Faber & Faber, London.

Roberts, I. (1975) *Discharged from Hospital*. Royal College of Nursing Study of Nursing Care Research Project, London.

Saunders, C. (1972) *Care of the Dying*. Nursing Times Publication, Basingstoke.

Saunders, C. (1978) *The Management of Terminal Disease*. Edward Arnold, London.

Skeet, M. (1978) *Home from Hospital*. Macmillan, London.

Skeet, M. (Comp.) (1981) *Discharge Procedures – Practical Guidelines for Nurses*, Nursing Times Publication, Basingstoke.

Thompson, I. (1980) *Dilemmas of dying – A Study in the Ethics of Terminal Care*. Edinburgh University Press, Edinburgh.

Tschudin, V. (1991) (3rd. ed) *Counselling Skills for Nurses*. Baillière Tindall, London.

Wilson-Barnett, J. (1979) *Stress in Hospital: Patient's Psychological Reactions to Illness and Health Care*. Churchill Livingstone, Edinburgh.

Wilson-Barnett, J. (ed.) (1983) Patient teaching. *Recent Advances in Nursing*. 6 Churchill Livingstone, Edinburgh.

Chapter 10
Creating a high morale within the team

Morale affects the stability of any group, the way in which the members of that group get on together and the way in which their activities are carried out, so if the nursing team is to be effective its morale must be high.

The morale of the patients depends very much on that of the nursing team and since the patients' state of mind whilst in hospital may control their rate of recovery (Revans, 1964) a ward environment conducive to good health is essential. As the leader of the nursing team the ward sister or charge nurse sets the tone, and therefore must be a skilled leader and able organizer. Within the ward this can be extremely difficult as it is an ever changing environment, so the sister or charge nurse has to continually strive to maintain the morale.

Developing good morale within a ward may not be an easy task. There are numerous factors which can contribute to good morale, and as many if not more that can reduce morale. Figure 10.1 shows some of the factors which can contribute to good morale. Figure 10.2 shows some of the factors which can contribute to poor morale within a ward. These figures are very generalized and do not attempt to describe all the factors

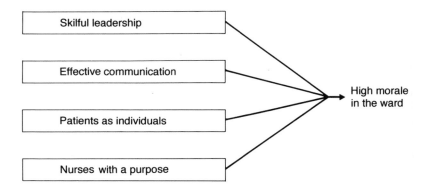

Fig. 10.1   Factors which help to create a high morale within the world.

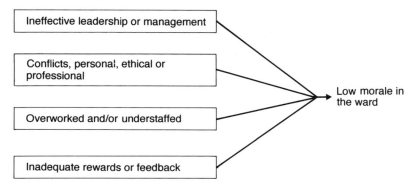

Fig. 10.2 Factors which may contribute to poor morale within the ward.

that may be involved but, rather, present some of the most common. Each situation has its own unique set of causative factors, dependent on the personalities of the individuals as well as on the group dynamics of the nursing team and others involved in the ward. The situation may also be affected by a patient or patient group. The problem of maintaining a high morale can be a difficult one as a result, and needs constant vigilance and assessment. Some of the factors that should be considered when thinking about morale are discussed in more detail now, to provide a starting point for nurses taking on a ward for the first time.

The reception given to the patients on admission to the ward will have an effect on their morale. If they are pleasantly and courteously welcomed, and if they sense that the nurses are concerned for them, their anxiety will be reduced and their confidence increased. On the whole patients are usually a sociable, friendly and sympathetic group of people who, if treated in the correct manner, will create a pleasant atmosphere and boost each other's morale. This is mentioned here for emphasis but is covered in more depth in Chapter 7.

If the nurses feel a sense of purpose within the ward and gain satisfaction in their work their morale should be high. They will feel a sense of purpose if the responsibility for patient care is delegated and they are held accountable for the care they give. Although the sister or charge nurse may feel that it is easier and quicker to do things rather than teach and delegate, it must be realized that by delegating to them the team members will be given an opportunity to give of their best. The nurses will feel that they are thought to be capable and trustworthy and this will help to build their self-confidence. In the ward where the sister or charge nurse effectively manages and delegates, the work will continue smoothly in her or his absence, with the ward properly organized and the patients well cared for.

Morale in the ward will be affected by the attitude of the more experienced members of the team to the less experienced. Those with more experience should be helpful and supportive and always approachable. If staff are made to feel welcome on first coming to the ward this, too, will help to maintain a good ward atmosphere. The various ways in which the members of the team communicate and relate to one another will affect the climate of the ward. If the right tone of voice, facial expression and eye contact are adopted by the senior staff this, too, will help to foster a good ward climate. This has been explained in Chapter 2.

A good rapport between team members should be encouraged, with a friendly but professional working relationship where everyone strives towards a high standard of patient care. If the group morale is high, each member will be more able to cope with stress and adversity. In periods when either the dependency of the patients is high above the normal level for that ward, or there are staff shortages or a rapid turnover of patients, the nursing team will respond well to these situations. They will give support and encouragement to one another, supported by the sister or charge nurse.

Each nurse must be aware of the team's objectives and therefore should appreciate her or his place in the total therapeutic plan. This applies to all members of the nursing team, whatever their grade, as well as the domestic and the clerical staff. The team members must each see the value of their own role and contribution and know what is expected of them. This will, to a great extent, depend upon how effectively the leadership role is carried out by the sister or charge nurse.

If the morale is to remain high each person needs to feel a sense of progress and be aware of how she or he is getting on in the ward. For student nurses this will come through placement assessments, for trained nurses through their annual appraisal and for the support workers and nursing auxiliaries through their annual progress report. This should, however be on-going and not only occur at the appraisal. Words of encouragement and praise should always be given when deserved, and thanks for work well done are always appreciated, whatever the grade or status of the person concerned.

Good communication and liaison between staff, patients and their relatives and other nursing departments and health care workers is vital, as emphasized in Chapter 2. This will affect morale within the ward. Principles taught in the college of nursing should be demonstrated in the ward. If not, the morale of the nurses in training will be affected as they will become confused, sensing conflict between their training and reality.

It is essential for the morale of the ward that all the staff are kept up-to-date and aware of what is happening within the ward, the unit, the hospital and the health district. Regular ward meetings, communications boards and communication books all have a part to play in helping to keep everyone informed and are discussed at length in Chapter 2.

If the sister or charge nurse provides effective leadership, which must include supervision and good communication, the nurse should feel happy and secure within the ward or department. The ward will be an efficiently run organization with each team member carrying out her or his role correctly and safely. The leadership role of the ward sister or charge nurse is now defined more fully.

Leadership

'A leader is a member of a group or organization who outstandingly influences the activities of the members of the group and plays a central role in defining goals and in determining the ideology of the organization. The leader has more influence on the group than the group has on the leader.' (Argyle, 1972).

Assessing the effectiveness of a leader is often easier when looking at the end results, thus a ward with high team morale and happy patients who are making good progress, would indicate effective leadership.

Qualities which make a good leader include a belief in the group's aims and objectives, effective communication, the ability to take in messages from the environment which will influence the instructions the leader gives, and the ability to keep the emotional climate constant through many changing situations. For example, in any ward there is frequent change amongst the personnel – student nurses allocated for a set number of weeks and some doctors change every six months – so each new person will need introducing to the ward and the members of the team and feel involved from the beginning and not left to feel an outsider. If they are not integrated properly they could prove a disrupting influence. A word of welcome and reassurance from the ward sister or charge nurse will ensure that the good ward climate is not adversely affected.

An able leader must also possess specific abilities in her or his speciality, for example, a sister or charge nurse in an oncology ward will need to know the side effects of chemotherapy and how to manage these from a nursing point of view.

The competent leader shows confidence in her or his own abilities but is not over-confident, and is able to take decisions speedily but effectively and enlist help if necessary. The leader must also be consistent, dependable and sensitive to the needs of others, that is, patients and staff. Leadership qualities should include:

- Intelligence and good judgement
- Insight and imagination
- The ability to accept responsibility
- A sense of humour
- A well-balanced personality
- A sense of justice.

These qualities were determined by the observation of several people in leadership situations. All points are of equal importance (Smith, 1958) and still apply today.

Additional leadership qualities include the power to communicate, an ability to supervise, plan and coordinate and to make appropriate and timely decisions. To successfully show these qualities, the ward sister or charge nurse must be able to delegate authority and responsibility for care to others, and give support and encouragement. The good leader passes on knowledge and skills and is able to teach and give guidance.

Not all leaders possess all these qualities to the same degree, but ward sisters and charge nurses need to have most of them. Leadership can be formal and informal, being specific to any given situation.

It was described in Chapter 1 how research in social science has contributed to our understanding of leaders. Leaders who are considerate of their subordinates and responsive to their needs produce better results. Similarly, those who place high importance on getting the job done, and who ensure that the environment and facilities are available to achieve that end, make better leaders. Frequently, leaders are described using the classification used by Lewin, Lipitt and White (1939), namely, as autocratic, democratic or laissez-faire. It is worth looking at the characteristics of each of these in some detail, applying them to the leader of the nursing team, as it helps to understand why the democratic leader is more able to produce a ward environment where a high morale is prevalent.

Autocratic leader

The autocratic leader is stern and strict. She or he is the type of leader who does not encourage ideas and questions but says 'on this ward the nurses know their place. I make the decisions as I have had far more experience than they have'. If suggestions are made they will be conveniently forgotten. The autocratic leader gives orders, determines group policy without consulting the group, discusses only immediate plans and not the future. This type of leader remains aloof from the group and will criticize individual group members in front of the others. The autocratic leader is the person who makes nurses afraid.

The autocratic leader expects all decisions to be made by herself or himself, discouraging other members of the nursing team from making any decision relating to patient care or ward policy. In other words, the autocratic leader does not delegate. However, she or he will be heard to say that she or he is the only person who does anything in the ward. The autocrat tends to resent anyone but herself or himself having in-depth discussion with patients or their relatives, arguing that the newly qualified staff nurse has not enough experience.

In the ward with an autocratic leader the morale of the nursing team tends to be low; the team members show little interest in their work and no initiative, and do only what they have to do. The nurses feel unimportant, have no sense of responsibility and gain little satisfaction from their work. They tend to become dependent on the sister or charge nurse as she or he tells them everything they have to do, leaving no decisions for them to make. They are frightened to make decisions in the absence of the sister or charge nurse; the fear is based on a possible disagreement with that decision. The nurses also tend to seek the attention of the sister or charge nurse, expecting approval for all that they do. Subordinates may even vie with one another for the leader's favour. In the absence of the sister or charge nurse there is a tendency for some of the subordinates to release their pent-up feelings and act in an unprofessional manner. Many nurses soon leave an autocratic situation and therefore there are many comings and goings amongst the nursing team which, in itself, leads to instability and low morale. The patients in this type of ward feel ill at ease and are afraid to seek any information from the sister or charge nurse. Unfortunately, nurses experiencing this type of leadership often adopt the same attitude and this becomes self-perpetuating.

Laissez-faire leader

The laissez-fair leader does not lead at all. The nursing team is left to get on with the job and they feel that there is no one at the helm guiding, supporting and encouraging them. This leads to a lack of direction and a feeling of frustration. The nurses in the team feel that nobody cares how they perform and therefore they may lower their standards.

The sister or charge nurse distributes responsibility amongst the members of the team in a disorganized way and then abdicates all responsibility. However, she or he will maintain that 'on this ward I delegate to my nurses to give them the experience they need'. However, the sister or charge nurse is not involved and does not follow up what has been delegated. For example, if the person who normally does the off-duty rota is sick it does not get done; stocks often run out if the responsibility for them is not delegated to a specific person; nurses' progress reports are not completed on time.

Communication between the team members is inadequate, mainly because the leader is not involved, and vital information does not get passed on or is missed altogether. The team members feel that they do not know what is going on in the ward. They muddle on, aware that they have no leader.

In this type of ward the patients feel insecure and are very aware of a lack of information about their treatment and progress.

Democratic leader

In the ward with a democratic sister or charge nurse decisions are made only after discussion with the ward nursing team. The democratic leader gives praise or criticism as indicated, but usually to the group as a whole. If there is a need to discuss a disciplinary matter this is done by taking the nurse aside, and never discussing the matter in front of one's colleagues.

The democratic sister or charge nurse is an approachable person who is always willing to listen to suggestions and constructive criticism from members of the team. She or he ensures that each nurse coming to the ward is aware of the work of the ward, the idiosyncrasies of the ward, what is expected of her or him, and the part she or he plays in the ward team. Any newcomer is made to feel a part of that team, and all the nurses are aware of the policies and procedures for that ward.

In the absence of the sister or charge nurse things continue to run smoothly and efficiently. Each person shows concern for her or his subordinates. Therefore, because they feel secure in the situation, the staff nurses, enrolled nurses, or senior student nurses, will show concern for the well-being of the student nurses, support workers and auxiliary nurses working with them.

The trained nurses will take pride in teaching the student nurses and help them to increase their self-confidence. The democratic ward sister or charge nurse provides an atmosphere of emotional security, acting as a catalyst, holding the group together at all times, even when not present. Within the group the more skilful workers are looked on as an asset, but knowledge and information is pooled for the benefit of all the members. There is no indication of 'one-upmanship', where one nurse may find out certain information about a patient and then divulge it at an opportune moment in front of her or his colleagues. The nurse shares this knowledge for the good of the patient. The democratic sister or charge nurse is always alert to the needs of the staff and constructively counsels individuals towards personal and professional development.

In the democratic situation discipline is not ignored; it is maintained through the team members' respect for each other and value for one another's contribution. They take a pride in their work and make every effort to ensure that the ward runs smoothly and efficiently at all times. Often the 'problem' nurse responds positively in this type of ward.

The patients on this ward are well-informed, comfortable and secure and have confidence in the care they are receiving.

The Dos and Don'ts for good leadership

Do:

- Maintain consistent attitude
- Set a good example and be professional
- Organize your work well
- Plan ahead
- Communicate effectively
- Delegate effectively
- Always be available and approachable
- Show confidence in the team
- Get to know each team member
- Allow each nurse to use her or his initiative
- Praise and thank
- Ask rather than command
- Admit when wrong
- Always find time to listen
- Be receptive to differing points of view
- Find out all the facts
- Criticize constructively
- Inform each team member of her or his progress
- Create a questioning environment
- Ensure that the staff know they can count on your support
- Allow time for a report and review of the care prescribed.

Don't:

- Belittle
- Criticize in front of patients or staff
- Criticize destructively
- Take team members for granted
- Favour certain team members
- Constantly check up
- Interrupt work

- Take one nurse from one area to another – approach the appropriate nurse
- Be over-familiar with the staff
- Delegate, then do the job yourself.

Other factors affect the morale and climate of the ward. These include giving each team member a sense of responsibility and commitment, the way change is implemented by the sister or charge nurse, and the way the sister or charge nurse disciplines the staff.

Ensuring a sense of responsibility and commitment

All team members must be aware of the part they play in the total therapeutic plan for the ward and that their contribution to patient care is of value. They will feel a part of the team if they are properly orientated to the ward and this is discussed in Chapter 11.

Another way of ensuring a commitment from each member of the team is to give each one their own specific area of responsibility for the total running of the ward. The ward sister or charge nurse can delegate certain aspects of ward organization to each nurse, but must be prepared to supervise and coordinate these activities, and if necessary, train the nurse to do the job. Many things can be delegated in this manner.

Implementing change

It is in human nature to resist change as all changes bring insecurity. Unfortunately, many newly appointed sisters and charge nurses tend to try to change things straight away, and this alienates the staff who feel threatened by having a new leader. The suggestion of change increases their insecurity even more.

Before attempting to change anything it is essential that the confidence and support of all staff is obtained and this will take time and effort by the sister or charge nurse. It is also important to obtain the ideas of the team members and build on these.

Whenever change is contemplated, whatever it is, before embarking on the change full discussion with all the staff involved must take place. Time must be set aside for those involved to ask questions and talk through their fears and anxieties. Reassurance needs to be given that if the proposed changes are not satisfactory there is no reason why the original system should not be used again. Before implementing any change at all the whole team must believe the principles are right and be prepared to work towards them.

Once the new changes have been adopted discussion must continue, with time being set aside to assess how things are progressing and whether the changes have been beneficial or not. If it is considered that no improvement has been gained the team might feel that it would be better for all to continue as before.

Guiding and disciplining

Although it is not an easy part of the sister's or charge nurse's function, it is necessary on occasions to give guidance and also to deal with disciplinary matters (see Chapter 1). Dealing with an incident is never a pleasant task and the way in which it is done is important if ward and individual morale are to be maintained. It should be done privately, as soon as possible after the incident has occurred and never in front of patients or colleagues. It is most important that the sister or charge nurse has all the relevant facts which are put to the nurse. The nurse must then have an opportunity to put forward her or his side of the situation. It might be that the nurse is being criticized for not carrying out a procedure correctly. It may, however, be demonstrated by the nurse that the correct equipment to carry out the procedure is not available on the ward, or the nurse might have been expected to perform a procedure for which adequate instruction had not been given.

If new staff, or student nurses are not living up to expectations, this must be discussed with them at an early stage in their allocation to the ward, rather than when they are given either their placement progress assessment or their annual appraisal. This will give the nurse concerned an opportunity to make an effort to improve. It also gives the nurse an opportunity to discuss any problems encountered which may be affecting her or his standard of work. It is morally wrong for the nurse to find that her or his standard of work is not good enough when she or he is faced with a written report or appraisal.

When reprimanding or disciplining members of staff it is also important to pay attention to their strong characteristics. Once a person has been disciplined this should be quickly followed up with a pleasant approach to enable the member of staff to feel that the sister or charge nurse still has confidence in them.

Where the sister or charge nurse emphasizes good communication and concern for staff, learners appreciate the good atmosphere and often want to return to work in the ward or department once qualified.

Topics for discussion

1. A newly appointed ward sister becomes aware that the morale of the staff on her ward is not as good as she feels it could be. At first she feels it only by instinct, but gradually picks up other cues such as a general reluctance to cooperate when changes in off-duty are discussed.

How could this sister pick up other clues as to the level of morale amongst the team of nurses?

Discuss three interventions she may use to try to raise the level of morale.

References and Recommended Reading

Argyle, M. (1972) *The Psychology of Interpersonal Behaviour*. Pelican Original, Harmondsworth.

Brown, J.A.C. (1954) *The Social Psychology of Industry*. Pelican Original, Harmondsworth.

Kron, T. (1987) *The Management of Patient Care – Putting Leadership Skills to Work*. W.B. Saunders & Co. London, Toronto, Philadelphia.

Lewin, K; Lipitt, R. & White, R.K. (1939) 'Patterns of aggressive behaviour in experimentally created social climates' *Journal of Social Psychology*, **10**, 271–99.

Orton, H. (1980) *Ward Learning Climate*. Royal College of Nursing, London.

Revans, R.W. (1964) *Standards for Morale: Cause and Effect in Hospitals*. Oxford University Press, Oxford.

Schurr, M. (1968) *Leadership and the Nurse*. The English Universities Press Ltd, London.

Smith, M. (1958 – reprint) *An Introduction to Industrial Psychology*. (5th ed.) Cassell, London.

Chapter 11
Teaching in the ward

Teaching and training are two very significant aspects of the sister's or charge nurse's role, carrying with it a commitment to train all members of the nursing team – staff nurses, enrolled nurses, student nurses, support workers, nursing auxiliaries – and patients and their relatives. There is also the need for the ongoing education of sisters and charge nurses.

Creating a learning environment

Factors which affect the learning environment of the ward are many but the most important are:

- The attitude of the sister or charge nurse to learning within the ward
- The awareness of all trained nurses of their teaching responsibility
- A high morale
- Emphasis on patients' needs rather than those of the ward
- Actively encouraging questions.

To create an environment which is meaningful and conducive to learning, the attitude of the sister or charge nurse is crucial. In her research, Orton (1980) has shown that student nurse learning is more likely to take place in wards with high student orientation, the sister or charge nurse emphasizing their learning needs, ensuring that they become a part of the ward team and meeting their emotional needs. She also highlighted that patient well-bring and student well-being are inextricably linked. The sister or charge nurse must, however, be seen to give high priority to the teaching and training of all grades of staff. Staff members who feel that priority is given to this aspect of the job will be more responsive and better motivated towards their work, which in turn will have a direct bearing on the standard of patient care. They will also be more aware of their own teaching responsibilities and this will help to create and maintain a learning environment. Orton (1980), Ogier (1981) and Fretwell (1982) have all conducted research which shows that the sister or charge nurse is the key person in creating a good word learning environment. In her study, Reid (1985) found that less than 50 per cent of the ward staff's time was devoted to direct patient care and that trained staff spent very little time teaching, but those sisters who deployed the staff most effectively provided the best learning environment.

If emphasis is placed on this aspect of the trained nurses' role the staff will be more likely to assist new nurses to become properly orientated to the ward. They will also be prepared to work with, and supervise the learners at the bedside. The attitude that it is quicker and easier to do a thing oneself is not conducive to learning, so the sister or charge nurse must also be prepared to spend time with all members of the team and also be ready to delegate. The attitude of the medical staff within the ward will also have an effect on the learning environment.

Maintaining a high morale within the team will enhance the learning environment. This will ensure that the team members, especially student nurses and those new to the ward, feel that support is readily given by the more senior nurses. Senior staff will also be more willing to spend time with the less experienced team members, working with them giving guidance and supervision.

By emphasizing the patients' needs rather than those of the ward, the needs of the nurses will also be catered for. This indicates that in an environment where patients' needs are met the attitude of caring embraces staff as well as patients. Orton (1980) observed that a ward that was highly orientated to the learning needs of the students exhibited a combination of teamwork, consultation and an awareness by the sister or charge nurse of the needs of subordinates.

Actively encouraging questions and providing the answers will encourage learning in a very positive way, helping nurses to learn through understanding. Nurses need to be stimulated to discuss and question nursing practice and be able to test their understanding and learning. This occurs if questions are invited. It does not necessarily mean that the sister or charge nurse has to have all the answers, provided she or he is prepared to obtain them. It is impossible for one person to know everything but answers can often be obtained from the team provided there is a good team spirit. Once confidence has been gained the nurses can be encouraged to ask questions of other health workers and paramedical staff such as doctors, physiotherapists and pharmacists.

The sister or charge nurse must appreciate that many nurses are afraid to ask questions as they are frightened that they may appear foolish in front of their colleagues, therefore they carry on in ignorance. It is possible to give the nurses an opportunity to ask questions without feeling self-conscious by asking 'Do you all understand? It is rather difficult to grasp. I had problems at first.' or 'Does anyone know what that means?' or 'Perhaps there are some of you who do not fully understand that.' Questions should never be directed to a particular person unless the sister or charge nurse is sure that the person is able to cope without feeling threatened.

Ways of teaching and learning in the ward

Teaching and learning in the ward takes place in a variety of ways and there are many opportunities for teaching in the clinical field:

- Acting as role model for trained nurses and students
- Orientating *all* new members of staff to the ward and their role
- Demonstrating skills and then supervising the student
- Encouraging a questioning atmosphere
- Sharing experiences through ward discussions, forums, seminars, and the effective use of the 'handover'
- Discussing patients with the nurses, doctors and other health care workers
- Planned teaching programmes involving trained nurses, doctors, other health care workers
- Nursing round of patients with student nurses
- Planning for senior students to work alongside the sister or charge nurse to learn aspects of ward management
- Involvement in medical rounds of patients
- Enabling nurses to visit appropriate outpatient clinics
- Enabling nurses to accompany patients to theatre, X-ray department, isotope department and any other appropriate departments, and on home visits
- Demonstrations by other health care workers, e.g. physiotherapist, occupational therapist
- Use of visual aids, for example diagrams, charts, tapes and slides, models and graphical displays on noticeboards
- Availability of, for example, books, journals, articles and pro- grammed texts.

Sisters and charge nurses act as role models to each member of their nursing team for their whole span of duty. This is one of the most effective ways of teaching, so the behaviour of the sister or charge nurse must be exemplary at all times.

The sister's or charge nurse's presence provides stability and she or he must try to be constant and never moody. The way in which patients and relatives are approached and spoken to, and the way in which information is imparted to them is in itself a learning experience, especially if the nurse concerned with the patient's care is included. If the sister or charge nurse demonstrates the importance of talking with all the patients during the day, allowing an opportunity to assess the patients and giving them a chance to ask questions, this will serve as an example to other members of staff as she or he will be seen to attach high priority to contact with patients. During the day there are many chances to teach on the ward those aspects of care which cannot be taught in the classroom. This will include such things as talking to patients, assessing their needs and allaying their anxieties, the administration of drugs, supporting patient's relatives by listening to them and talking to relatives on the telephone.

Time spent discussing and then demonstrating a skill, or talking about the best way of coping with certain aspects of care, such as preventing the development of pressure sores in a paralysed patient, is very worthwhile and meaningful. Sisters and charge nurses must also be prepared to delegate the responsibility for the total care of patients to members of the team, as long as they are sure of the capabilities of the nurse to whom they are delegating. By allowing nurses to increase their experience in this way learning is encouraged. The delegation of care to student nurses, however, will always be under the supervision of a trained nurse. This helps to increase the confidence of the nurses in their own abilities, and learning occurs through experience. The handover period is a time when nursing care can be discussed and evaluated, explanations given, questions encouraged and the importance of all aspects of care can be stressed. Topics such as pain control, care of bladder and bowels, the reaction of a patient to admission to hospital and loss of independence, mobilization of patients, care and support of the terminally ill, the ethical issues raised by resuscitation and other issues which cause nurses anxiety are some areas worthy of discussion. Planning for the discharge of patients can be beneficially discussed at the handover. The whole team is involved in this valuable learning experience.

Often, when discussing the teaching role of the trained nurse, it is considered that teaching can only occur in a formal setting, but this is a very small part of the teaching which takes place in the ward. To many trained nurses the thought of teaching formally can be very daunting, but initial nervousness may be overcome by having small groups of two or three students.

Although it can be difficult to make time for this form of teaching in a busy ward this can be achieved if carefully thought out and planned ahead. Nurse teachers, doctors and other health care workers can be included as well as the trained nurses within the ward team. The afternoon overlap, where it occurs, may be used for this purpose.

A joint teaching programme with a neighbouring ward of a similar speciality, or on a unit basis, might be a worthwhile consideration. A programme could be planned and students chosen to attend or, alternatively, nurses allowed to choose which sessions would be most beneficial to them at their stage of training. An example is given in Table 11.1. Teaching can take place in a quiet place away from the ward, or, with the patient's permission, at the bedside, involving the patient in the discussion. This will help to make learning more meaningful.

The nurse responsible for a patient can be encouraged to discuss the nursing care which has been planned based on the physical and psychological needs. The reasons for a particular plan of care may be discussed and the effect of that care evaluated. This type of discussion will help nurses to be more analytical and critical of their performance and enable them to appreciate different approaches to patient care and the fulfilment of patients' needs.

Articles from nursing journals which relate to the art of nursing as well as the clinical speciality, and up-to-date textbooks provide valuable

Table 11.1 Example of a formal teaching programme.

Wards 3 and 4. Medically Orientated Teaching Programme.

Sun 3rd June	The Nursing Problems Associated with Bedrest. Staff Nurse Pearce
Wed 6th June	Rehabilitation of a Patient After a Cerebro-vascular Accident Sister Palmer
Sun 10th June	Overcoming Incontinence in the Elderly. Staff Nurse Merrill
Wed 13th June	Caring for the Patient with Severe Breathlessness Staff Nurse Lynch
Sun 17th June	Caring for the Patient with Chest Pain Sister Jones
Wed 20th June	Caring for the Severely Anaemic Patient Staff Nurse Davies
Sun 24th June	Effective Pain Control Sister Palmer
Wed 27th June	The More Commonly Used Drugs – Their Actions and Side Effects Staff Nurse Ryan

reference in the ward. Diagrams and charts also serve a similar purpose. These must all be readily available and not locked away if they are to be of any value. A well planned notice board can be very effective but quick to prepare.

It may be difficult to obtain books because of the expense involved, but with the help of the unit nurse manager this obstacle may be overcome since funds are often available for this purpose. Well-motivated staff nurses or enrolled nurses may be willing to produce charts or diagrams as teaching aids.

The ward sister or charge nurse has a responsibility for teaching and training all levels of nursing staff. She must have an understanding of the working of the professional boards and of the courses available for student nurses to attain registration as well as those for post-registration education.

United Kingdom Central Council (UKCC) and the National Boards

The Nurses, Midwives and Health Visitors Act of 1979 established the UKCC for Nurses, Midwives and Health Visitors, and National Boards for the four parts of the United Kingdom.

UKCC

Principle functions are to:

(1) Establish and improve standards of education and training and professional conduct.
(2) Maintain a 'live' professional register (consisting of practising nurses, midwives and health visitors) and control admission to the register.

Periodic registration has been introduced in order to maintain the register. It is hoped that before 1995 courses will be mandatory for nurses re-entering the profession after a break, as it now is for midwives. When re-registering, nurses will be required to produce evidence of continuing education.

National Boards

The four boards are concerned with courses of training at basic and post-basic level, and for ensuring that the standard and content of all courses meet the requirements of the Central Council. They are also required to promote improved concepts and methods of training, based on the needs of society.

'Project 2000'

Project 2000 was set up by the UKCC in 1986 to review the professional preparation of Nurses, Midwives and Health Visitors in order to prepare for the health care needs of society in the 1990s and beyond. It has since been approved as the new system of nurse training. Project 2000 is based on health promotion, prevention and early detection of disease, not solely on the curative aspects of care. This approach is centred on the individual, the family and the community and is undertaken in colleges of nursing and midwifery with established links with colleges of higher education. At present the system is running concurrently with the traditional system of training but will eventually take its place. Midwifery training is not yet part of Project 2000 training.

Project 2000 has achieved the introduction of a single level of registered nurse at diploma level, who must be an analytical, knowledgeable and independent practitioner, able to practice in hospital and the community. The position of the second-level or enrolled nurse is safeguarded but active encouragement is offered to enrolled nurses wishing to convert to first-level nurses, and there are a variety of ways this can be achieved.

Training is firmly based on an educationally determined curriculum. The training period is three years. The first 18 months, called the Common Foundation Programme, is a general introduction to nursing and concentrates on the nature of nursing. It is based on the biological, sociological and behavioural sciences, and ethical, environmental, legal and political issues are examined. Health promotion and disease prevention are both given high priority.

The second 18 months, known as the Branch Programme, concentrates on preparation to practice in a particular branch of nursing – mental health, mental handicap, nursing adults or nursing children (see Fig 11.1). The nurse is expected to apply the broad principles and skills attained in the Common Foundation Programme in assessing, planning, implementing and evaluating care, and to develop knowledge, competence and expertise in the care of patients in his or her chosen speciality. This includes an elective period to study a specific aspect of the branch being studied.

Strict criteria are laid down which must be met by wards and departments before they can be considered suitable training areas for Project 2000 students. Some of the following are expected:

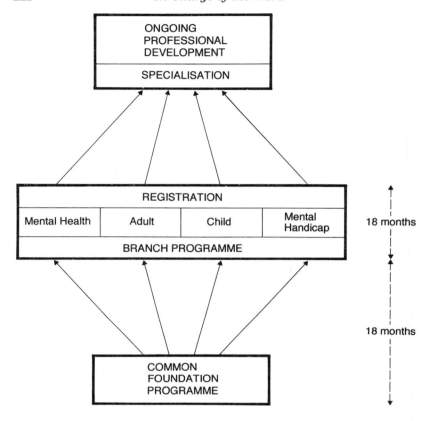

Fig. 11.1 Project 2000 Structure.

- Adequate preparation of all trained staff for the supervision and assessment of Project 2000 students and a total understanding of supernumerary status
- A progressive and innovative environment
- The continuous evaluation of nursing practice
- Evidence that nursing practice is based on current research findings
- Adequate staffing levels to provide realistic supervision and support for the student nurses
- Effective teaching and learning strategies with a commitment by the staff for teaching and self-development
- Effective management
- Good channels of communication.

Supernumerary status

During the Project 2000 training programme student nurses gain their practical experience where their educational programme requires. They are supernumerary to manpower needs for most of the clinical placements, both in the community and in hospital, i.e. they are not part of the service commitment until the middle of the third year of training. Supernumerary means that the students, although part of the ward team, are not included in the normal staff complement and, at all times, are given the opportunity to observe and participate in nursing care activities under close supervision. They need to be able, with continuous support and supervision, to apply theory learned in the academic centre. At least 50 per cent of the time will be spent in the clinical environment. Once part of the rostered service, i.e. included in the manpower needs of the clinical area, the students will be expected to participate in nursing decisions and care relating to patients, but will still be supervised. Payment throughout the three-year course is by a non-means-tested bursary.

It has been established that the ward sister or charge nurse has a commitment to teach and train registered and enrolled nurses, student nurses, support workers and auxiliary nurses. Each group will be considered in turn as the needs and expectations of each will vary.

Staff nurses and enrolled nurses

If the sister or charge nurse takes the time to arrange an orientation programme for all newly appointed trained nurses this should help them to evolve into conscientious and reliable members of the team, ensuring that the ward runs smoothly in the absence of the sister or charge nurse. This will only happen, however, if support and guidance is also given. An orientation programme could be planned to include those topics covered in Chapter 3.

The aims of all trained nurses are to be safe practitioners and to assist in the training of student nurses. During training they will have been educated to give a high standard of care and the significance of maintaining these high standards once qualified should be impressed upon them. All trained nurses must be encouraged to make use of every teaching opportunity available to them. It is essential to insist that whenever possible a trained nurse works with a student so that the learner nurse is taught at the bedside whilst performing nursing care. It is undesirable and often unsafe for one student nurse to be taught by another.

On first joining the ward team all trained nurses must know what is expected of them. They will need to know how to act when in charge of the ward for a span of duty and must also understand their role when not in charge so that conflicts between trained members of the team can be avoided. This is the responsibility of the sister or charge nurse. It is also important that the sister or charge nurse identifies the nurse who is new to the ward or speciality, or who is recently qualified so that support and guidance are given by all the trained members of the ward team.

In order that recently qualified staff nurses gain the experience necessary to organize the ward there must be a willingness to involve them in the management of the ward. This will only be effective if the sister or charge nurse delegates and gives them the authority and responsibility to make decisions and take certain action. In this way confidence and experience are gained. This experience should include talking with and listening to patients' relatives and attending doctors' rounds. Opportunity should also be given to liaise with other departments, order supplies and plan duty rotas. The writing of progress assessment reports for student nurses, support workers and auxiliary nurses is important experience.

Much of the information required by the newly appointed sister or charge nurse listed in Chapter 3 will be required by the newly appointed trained nurse, but may vary slightly from hospital to hospital and from ward to ward. Check lists are of value to the nurse, and act as an aide-mémoire.

Once properly orientated into the management aspects of the ward the newly trained nurses must be introduced to their teaching responsibilities. They may also have other learning needs related to the nursing speciality, especially if it is a new experience. In other instances it will be necessary for the nurse to learn about the medical or surgical techniques and special procedures used, together with the associated nursing care.

Student nurses

Student nurses in wards and departments may be in a state of conflict, though this is now lessening with the implementation of Project 2000. As nurses they are part of the nursing team and have an obligation to care for the patients but they are also students in a learning situation. As students they must be aided in their training by being given appropriate practical experience in wards and departments where they are conscious of guidance and support from the trained nurses. This is vital if they are to develop into caring, conscientious and dependable registered nurses. As maturing adults in a work environment they need to be able to develop self respect, to use their initiative and to think and act like adults. It is therefore essential that the sister or charge nurse treats them as adults. They will then respond in a positive manner. They will also be treated with respect by the other trained nurses in the team.

Nurses always state that learning is more meaningful in the ward as it is patient-centred, thus enabling them to relate theory to practice. It is essential that they gain as much experience and knowledge as possible during each ward and departmental allocation to help them to increase their self-confidence and become skilled practitioners. The best way to gain confidence and skill is to obtain sound practical experience and theoretical knowledge.

Practical experience is also essential so that a sense of achievement can be gained but this will depend on how that experience is obtained. If the student nurse is given the responsibility of caring for a group of patients with a trained nurse, the students will feel secure, develop new skills and become more confident, learning to assess priorities for care and plan and care for individual patients. They will also feel that they can use their initiative. Through participating in rehabilitation, relief of pain, successful resuscitation or assisting a patient to die peacefully, the student nurse will gain a sense of achievement. As long as the nurse feels that support and guidance is readily available, the correct practical experience will help the nurse to make decisions in a mature and objective way but, at the same time remaining sensitive and caring, responsive to the needs of the patients and their relatives.

When nurses are allocated to patients and student nurses work under the guidance of a trained nurse, those who are less experienced should have the chance to carry out duties and procedures that are the prerogative of the senior team members in wards organized on the lines of task allocation, thus increasing their skills. These skills will include observing and assisting with the administration of drugs, lumbar puncture, chest aspiration, dressing wounds, the commencement of intravenous infusion and so forth. Once the junior nurses have absorbed what they have observed, they must be allowed to participate with supervision from a senior nurse until they become proficient. Participation is important to increase dexterity in carrying out a procedure, such as the administration of drugs. If the nurse always acts as the observer and does not handle ampoules and containers, dexterity will not be achieved.

While the less experienced students are developing their procedural skills, the trained nurses and senior nurses who are closely involved in the bedside nursing of the patient, must encourage the less experienced nurses to develop their nursing care skills. The senior nurses have the opportunity to pass on to the less experienced members of the team the theoretical as well as practical aspects of total nursing care.

On first arriving at the ward or department the student nurses will sense quickly whether there is a good learning atmosphere. This will be perceived through the reception received on first coming to the ward: whether they are expected, if made to feel welcome and introduced to the other staff, if shown around and their duties explained. A letter of introduction received beforehand will help them feel they are expected on the ward (see Fig. 11.2). Support will be achieved if the new learner is attached to a trained nurse with whom she or he works, especially during the early weeks of the allocation. This will involve careful planning of the duty rotas, although if the nurse is supernumerary it should not create a problem. The trained nurse, acting as a clinical supervisor or mentor, can then orientate the student to the new learning environment, introduce him or her to new colleagues and patients, and explain the pattern of the patients' and nurses' day and what is expected or her or him.

The mentor should perform all the interviews, the first during week one of the nurse's allocation. This may include:

● Ascertaining the stage of training reached by the student
● Ascertaining past experience of nursing and the speciality
● Assessing learning needs and expectations with the nurse
● Identifying fears and anxieties and how these may be overcome
● Setting plans of action to meet the identified learning needs i.e. skills and knowledge
● Discussing the learning opportunities
● Explaining the limits of the nurse's responsibility for patient care.

Later, progress interviews may include:

● Assessing the nurse's progress
● Discussing the learning opportunities in more detail
● Talking through any problems encountered
● Praising the nurse on her or his achievements.

A final interview should cover:

● Assessing the nurse's overall performance
● Discussing the formative assessment of the nurse's performance.

All the points mentioned above, however, should form an on-going interaction between nurse and mentor.

By having a trained nurse to relate to, the learner should feel less isolated and less stressed, making the allocation a more meaningful learning experience. In the mentor's absence, other trained nurses will be involved in the teaching programme and will be available to give help, supervision, guidance and support. By acting as mentors, all the trained nurses should gain more job satisfaction, be more aware of their responsibilities as a registered nurse, and keep themselves up to date

Blackwell General Hospital

Ward 30

30 July 1992

Dear Jane,

You will soon be coming to Ward 30 as part of your training programme. We hope that your stay will be enjoyable and the experience worthwhile and of value to you.

There will be many learning opportunities for you and all the staff will be most willing to help you gain the experience and knowledge and develop the practical skills you hope to achieve whilst with us.

As a temporary member of the team your presence will be valued, so do feel that you can contribute to discussions and make any constructive criticism you feel may improve patient care, or the experience of the student nurse. Also, if in doubt about anything at all, do not hesitate to ask.

The philosophy of the ward is:

To give the highest quality of care, adopting a holistic approach to each patient, treating each one as an individual person with unique needs.

The nurse works in partnership with the patient and his or her family, helping them through the stages of illness and to accept limitations and disabilities. This will involve promoting independence within each patient's limitations, or helping him or her to a peaceful and dignified death. Continuity of care is of paramount importance and so is the provision of information which the patient and his or her family are able to understand.

During your placement your mentor will be . . . . who will be responsible for supervising, guiding and supporting you, completing your initial and progress interviews and on-going assessment. The other team members will be willing to support and help you and you are free to turn to them for advice if you wish.

With best wishes from the staff of Ward 30.

Signed

. . . .

Fig. 11.2 An example of an introductory letter to a student nurse.

Introduces the student to the ward
Performs first, intermediate and final interviews
Identifies learning needs
Identifies fears and anxieties and ways of allaying these
Source of support and encouragement
Teacher   provides/identifies learning opportunities
               resource person
               role model
               demonstrates practical skills
               supervises practical skills
Supervisor
Assessor
Counsellor
Guide

Fig. 11.3 Summary of the mentor's role.

clinically and professionally. The mentor makes educational progress possible for the student nurse. The role of the nurse mentor is summarized in Figure 11.3. Ideally, students should always work with a trained nurse. This is not always possible, so the sister or charge nurse must supervise their work. The nurses must be aware that they will be expected to account for the care given by them and that their work will be reviewed, and care evaluated and replanned if necessary at a set time during the day. The fact that all care does not have to be completed by lunchtime may need stressing – many nurses often feel this is expected of them.

Learning opportunities

Learning opportunities are written statements of learning experience available on each ward for student nurses. They are based on the content and learning outcomes of the course curriculum and are founded on biological, sociological and behavioural sciences, together with health promotion and disease prevention as well as cure. Ethical, environmental, legal and political issues are also included. Learning opportunities are usually written by members of the ward team in conjunction with the academic supervisor or link teacher from the college of nursing. They are written in easily understood terminology and must be realistic and attainable (see Tables 11.2, 11.3 and 11.4).

If this information is readily available to each student nurse allocated to the ward, together with a profile of the ward, it will enable her to gain an awareness of what to expect from the allocation, enabling the student to make the best use of all the experience – skills, attitudes and knowledge – available to her.

Table 11.2 Learning opportunities based on the activities of daily living; some examples.

Personal safety and comfort
  e.g. applying principles of asepsis
Communication
  e.g. helping the patient with speaking difficulties
Breathing
  e.g. helping the patient adopt a suitable position
  administering oxygen therapy
Eating and drinking
  e.g. assisting the patient with meals
Personal hygiene and dressing
  e.g. assisting the patient to dress and undress
Mobilization
  e.g. lifting and moving the patient safely
Elimination
  e.g. assisting with bedpan/commode/toilet
Maintaining body temperature
  e.g. helping reduce elevated temperature to promote comfort
Dignity and sexuality
  e.g. allowing the patient to dress as he or she chooses
Working and playing
  e.g. helping the patient to pursue his or her interests within the constraints of illness and the ward
Sleeping
  e.g. helping to promote a restful atmosphere
Dying
  e.g. helping the patient to a peaceful and dignified death

The level of achievement required of the student will vary from one placement to another, i.e. with different stages of the student's training.

Ward profile

A profile of the ward describes the characteristics of the environment, the different staff members associated with the ward and the type of patients likely to be cared for. It serves to give the student new to the ward a thumbnail sketch of the ward to which she or he has been allocated. Facilities for patients, staff and student nurses are usually included (see Table 11.5).

In the ward student nurses will make the most of the learning opportunities if the qualified nurses make good use of the numerous teaching opportunities available and give guidance, support and supervision. It is essential that the learners are encouraged to discuss any new experiences and that any doubts are explained. For this to be effective,

Table 11.3   Examples of learning opportunities available in most wards.

Whilst allocated to Ward 30, you will have the opportunity to care for people of:

- Different racial and ethnic groups
- Different cultures and creeds
- Different age groups 16–85+ years
- Both sexes
- Varying levels of dependency – ranging from totally dependent to self-caring

Also people:

- Coping with sudden, acute illness
- Coping with a variety of disabilities
- Undergoing rehabilitation programmes
- Needing care for 24 hours or several weeks
- In hospital for the first time

You will have the opportunity to observe in others and then develop in yourself, skills associated with caring for people in ill-health:

- Caring skills e.g. empathizing
- Observation skills e.g. recording body temperature
- Communication skills e.g. listening
- Assessment skills e.g. assessing needs
- Behavioural skills e.g. adapting approach to individuals
- Organizational skills e.g. planning care and prioritizing
- Analytical skills e.g. evaluating care

however, the qualified nurses must be aware of each learner's previous experience and also their expectations.

It is imperative for the qualified nurses to assess whether the learning opportunities are being used by the students. This can be accomplished in several ways. The trained nurse, whilst working alongside the students, can observe them and talk to them during their day-to-day care of the patients. As well as on-going observation there is also explicit observation of certain aspects of care such as the demonstration of a skill or asking the nurse to assess a particular patient's needs. The opinion of the student nurse should also be encouraged to ascertain whether the learner feels that the learning opportunities are realistic. In-depth discussion from time to time during the nurse's ward allocation will be necessary to assess knowledge and attitudes. Attitudes can also be assessed day by day as the nurse relates to patients, their relatives, colleagues and other health care workers. They will also become apparent when the nurse is contributing to the discussions at the daily ward report or handover. These methods of assessing form part of the continuous assessment of student nurses.

Learning opportunities (see Tables 11.2, 11.3 and 11.4) can be

Table 11.4   Examples of learning opportunities in communication.

During your placement you will be able to observe the trained nurse involve the patient and family in post-illness education and then participate in these activities:
  For example:

- Teaching new skills   giving an injection
    monitoring blood sugar
- Providing dietary education
- Discussing methods of reducing stress
- Discussing methods of changing lifestyle
- Involving self-help groups

During your placement you will have an opportunity to observe the trained nurse communicating with different groups of people involved in the care of the patient, and be given the chance to develop your own communication skills.
  For example:

- Ward nursing team
- Medical team
- Physiotherapists
- Occupational therapists
- Speech therapists
- Social worker
- Pharmacist

Table 11.5   One example of a ward profile.

Ward 30

Ward is a 28-bedded mixed-sex ward, accommodating patients with varying degrees of ill-health requiring medical intervention.

The ward is divided into 6 four-bedded rooms, a two-bedded room and 2 single rooms. There are 10 toilets, a shower, 3 bathrooms and a patient hoist. There is a dayroom with television and video for use by the patients.

There is a resource room for use by all grades of nursing staff and a medical and nursing library on site.

The care team consists of:

2 sisters	3 consultant physicians
12 staff nurses	5 registrars
8 support workers	1 senior house officer
1 ward clerk	3 house officers

A social worker, physiotherapist, occupational therapist, speech therapist, dietician and community liaison nurse, all liaise with the nursing and medical teams.

Assessing, planning, implementing and evaluating care is based on Roper, Logan and Tierney's Activities of Living. The aim of care is to meet the physical, psychological, spiritual and social needs of the patients through an individualized approach to them.

displayed centrally or given to each learner as a handout during the preliminary interview. Good liaison with the college of nursing is vital when nurses in training are working on the ward. The sister or charge nurse must keep up-to-date with what is taught in the college and at what stage so that she or he knows what to expect of each learner. The importance of demonstrating within the ward the methods and principles taught in the college of nursing cannot be emphasized enough. Principles must not be compromised in practice as this will influence the training environment of the ward and will lead to a lowering of standards of care as well as creating conflicts for the nurses in training.

Continuous assessment

The National Boards have given nurse teaching establishments greater autonomy to develop curricula and set examinations, devolving the final written examination to them. Continuous theoretical assessment takes place through essay writing, projects, assignments and formal written examinations. All work produced by the student is assessed.

Clinical assessment is performed by suitably trained registered practitioners during each placement, both in the community and in hospital. The assessor, who is usually the student's mentor or supervisor, will assess skills, knowledge and attitudes whilst the student is participating in nursing activities. There are written required levels of achievement, based on the course curriculum, for each stage of training during the length of the course, and clear pass/fail criteria are laid down. There is an element of self-assessment by the student with regard to the goals set and achievement of learning outcomes.

During the first placement of the Common Foundation Programme the outcomes will be simple but, as the nurse progresses through the first 18 months towards the Branch Programme, the expected outcomes will become more complex, as knowledge and skills are attained. All work performed by the student is assessed, therefore the expected practical levels of achievement must be available to all students during each placement. These will have been identified in the learning opportunities available on every ward and department involved in nurse training, and in the nurse's personal progressive assessment booklet for each placement.

Throughout the period of training, the nurse is expected to perform to the satisfaction of her or his supervisors. The main advantages of continuous assessment are that the assessment is not dependent on one performance by the nurse, on one specific day, but is a judgement of the nurse's performance overall, and a more comprehensive range of skills can be covered. The nurse's performance is often more consistent, as the assessment is based on everything she or he does. Hopefully, learning and assessment become interchangeable, thus reducing anxiety.

Support workers

The support worker was included in the nursing structure and those of other professions allied to nursing, such as physiotherapy, occupational therapy, speech therapy and chiropody, in a bid to meet service needs in the light of demographic changes in the 1990s. The need for another helper escalated with the introduction of Project 2000 and supernumerary status, resulting in a need to look at a replacement workforce.

Many existing nursing auxiliaries have been given the opportunity to have their competency assessed, as well as recruiting men and women new to nursing to fulfil the support worker role. There is no barrier, such as age, gender or lack of academic attainment, to training, which is undertaken locally both on and off the job, within a National Framework of Vocational Qualifications (NVQs). Skills, knowledge and pre-arranged competencies and standards of performance, based on national standards, are achieved at the student's own pace. NVQs have five levels of achievement, and may become a means of being considered for entry to nurse training.

The title of this group of staff will vary from place to place. Their duties will vary from ward to ward depending on the speciality and the wish of the person in overall charge of the ward. The support worker's role is to support the professional – the registered practitioner – in the delivery of the highest standard of care, working under her or his supervision and being responsible to that person. The registered practitioner delegates to the support worker but remains accountable for the care given and the outcomes of that care. The registered nurse will also be responsible for on-the-job training of the support worker and, after having received appropriate training, for the assessment of competence. Duties currently undertaken by ward clerks, receptionists and orderlies might be considered part of the support worker's role.

With the introduction of the support worker role exercises are being undertaken to reassess the skill mix in wards and departments. When these are being undertaken it is vital that the ward sister or charge nurse is totally involved to ensure the quality of the professional nursing given to the patients is not compromised.

Nursing auxiliaries

In many hospitals nursing auxiliaries, once allocated to a ward or department may spend several years there giving reliable service and helping to form some stability. It is therefore of paramount importance that auxiliary nurses are introduced to their duties in an organized way, and that they are fully aware of their duties and what is expected of them. Proper orientation should ensure that the nursing auxiliary becomes a dependable member of the ward nursing team.

Unfortunately in some wards, some nursing auxiliaries are allowed to carry out duties which they are neither trained for and for which they would not receive protection if anything were to go wrong. In the event of an error the sister or charge nurse is responsible so it is vital that she or he ensures that new nursing auxiliaries know their duties and the consequences of undertaking work for which they have not been trained.

A good guide to the role of nursing auxiliaries is that the care they give to patients in hospital is the care that a relative might give to a patient being nursed at home. It is becoming necessary to give nursing auxiliaries job descriptions, which usually list the tasks that they may perform, such as making beds and bathing patients.

Many newly appointed nursing auxiliaries receive a period of training prior to working in the clinical areas. During this time basic nursing procedures are taught and practical demonstrations given. The role of the auxiliary is discussed and the relationship between that role and that of others in the team. Aspects of safety are explained, including fire, accident prevention, and the auxiliary's own safety with emphasis on areas such as lifting, disposal of excreta, and nursing patients with infectious diseases. Attitudes to patients, relatives and colleagues is also an important area which is covered.

Once in the practical situation the nursing auxiliaries will learn by the example of other members of the team. They will also begin to practice tasks taught during their training, becoming gradually more skilled. During the first few months it is recommended that nursing auxiliaries work under the close supervision of a senior nurse so that their performance can be assessed and corrections made as indicated. Auxiliaries new to the ward should never be left to 'muddle through' on their own since this is extremely dangerous. Neither should two auxiliaries be left to work together if this can be avoided. In some wards and departments it might be practical for the auxiliary to be given specific duties as in the case of a department, or the care of a group of preconvalescent or independent patients if in a ward, provided there is adequate supervision from a senior nurse.

If there is no training available for nursing auxiliaries, and, on joining the hospital they are allocated straight to the wards, the sister or charge nurse should formulate a plan of orientation so that the auxiliaries have an opportunity to become aware of their role and what is expected of them, to enable them to become safe and competent. This should take place over a period of time, during which the auxiliary should work under the supervision of a trained nurse. Once a realistic programme of orientation has been planned a specific trained nurse can be given the responsibility of orientating a particular auxiliary. The programme will include explanation and demonstration of basic nursing procedures which are then practised under supervision, explanation of what is expected of an auxiliary and how auxiliaries fit into the nursing team, attitudes to patients and relatives, and the prevention of accidents to patients, to oneself, and others.

Nursing auxiliaries also have on-going learning needs and, as well as learning from the example of others, will also learn from in-depth discussions at the handover, especially if allowed to participate. At this time they will develop insight into the needs of specific patients in the ward, as well as an understanding of the reasons behind certain decisions.

With the recent introduction of the support worker role there will be fewer nursing auxiliaries in the ward team. Some will opt to undertake the support worker training if they are suitable, others will be lost through natural wastage over a period of time. In the future the role may be phased out altogether once the support worker training programme is well established. Until then nursing auxiliaries need to feel that they are valuable members of the nursing team.

Professional development

Ward sisters and charge nurses have a responsibility for their own on-going education. This involves keeping up-to-date with changes both clinically and within the nursing profession. It also means keeping up-to-date with changes in policy and management principles and this can be achieved in several ways. Some of the more obvious ways are reading nursing journals and research publications, attending meetings of professional organizations and groups, and at unit meetings. Many hospitals have excellent library facilities with up-to-date books as well as a variety of both nursing and medical journals, supplying a wide range of knowledge. Developments in nursing research are being made constantly and sisters and charge nurses should be prepared to read research publications which are relevant to their clinical situation or which relate to nursing management. They should make every effort to understand the findings and be willing to implement them if they will enhance patient care (see Chapter 4).

There are other opportunities to keep up-to-date with changes within the profession and also clinical developments, and this is to take advantage of courses, study days and conferences, both locally and further afield. It should not be left to nurse managers to approach sisters and charge nurses, inviting them to make applications to attend study days and conferences but the sisters and charge nurses themselves should approach their managers if they feel it would be of value to attend. Following registration, there are many courses available to enable nurses to participate in their own professional and clinical development. Courses for other parts of the register may be taken, e.g. Registered Sick Children's Nurse, and there are a range of short courses and six-month courses approved by the National Boards which aim to give trained nurses an opportunity to increase their knowledge, understanding and experience in a chosen field.

Other approved courses are aimed at enhancing professional practice and development, such as understanding and applying research, teaching and assessing in clinical practice, and continuing care of dying patients and their families.

A registered nurse may wish to gain the Diploma in Nursing of the University of London, or the Diploma in Advanced Nursing Studies, or a health related degree, which may be taken on a full or part time basis. Professional organizations and trade unions also organize courses.

As well as the Open University courses, there are other distance learning and correspondence courses available to nurses. These include programmes for the conversion of the enrolled nurse, courses in 'managing care' and the diploma in nursing.

It is usually expected that either on or before appointment, sisters and charge nurses attend a recognized management course, or a course specifically aimed at preparing them for their new role.

Post-Registration Education and Practice Project

The UKCC is concerned that, once qualified, nurses continue to develop professionally, building on the process begun during basic education, so Post-Registration Education and Practice Project (PREPP) was set up. A framework is being developed so that, in the future, all qualified nurses – both first and second level – will be required to up-date themselves continually in order to meet the needs of clients and patients.

It is fundamentally important that continuing education relates to practice so that practitioners maintain a level of competence and standard of care acceptable to the profession. Every nurse, therefore, from commencing to ceasing practice, will be required to develop professionally. In the near future it will be a requirement that, before each periodic re-registration, evidence of professional learning and development, both practical and academic, is available. Practitioners will be required to keep a personal and professional development profile in order to be eligible to practice. This will almost certainly become a statutory requirement.

Credit Accumulation and Transfer Scheme

Courses and educational qualifications achieved prior to and since nurse training, may be accredited with Credit Accumulation and Transfer Scheme (CATS) points. These points are accumulative and can be used as a basis for further studies in higher education, e.g. Diploma and Degree courses.

Points are awarded for different courses, e.g. nurses registered since a certain date will be awarded 120 points whilst 60 points are accredited prior to that date. With 120 points the nurse may enter academic courses at level one. Other courses and possibly study days may be accredited with points, as may previous work undertaken, both academic and experiential.

It is not always easy to evaluate clinical experience but it is recognized that clinical experience plays a very important role when assessing a person's credit-worthiness for higher education.

It is essential that a balance between practical and academic experience is maintained and that practical experience is not underestimated. Short courses issue statements of attendance as proof of professional development. Certificates are given following the longer courses, and teaching and assessing in clinical practice is now usually incorporated in these courses to prepare trained nurses to assess student nurses, support workers and post-registration students in their own clinical environment.

Assessing the performance of all staff

The performance of all nurses in the ward or department is assessed by the sister or charge nurse or clinical manager at agreed times during their employment. Student nurses have a written progressive assessment by their mentor during each placement. This is in the form of a progressive assessment booklet. All trained nurses are assessed by the sister or charge nurse, usually annually, and support workers and nursing auxiliaries have an annual written report. The assessment of trained nurses takes the form of a development and performance review which identifies areas for development mutually agreed by appraiser and appraisee. The objectives of staff appraisal are set out in Chapter 1, but some tips as to how to conduct one are valuable too.

Any assessment or report on a member of staff must be completed objectively, and be seen as an opportunity to develop staff rather than to criticize them. Adequate time should be set aside to allow discussion of the assessment, which should be undertaken in a quiet place without interruption. If it is difficult to find somewhere quiet it may be necessary to move away from the working area.

When making an assessment it is vital to emphasize good qualities as well as those which need to be strengthened and improved upon. It is, however, good personnel management to discuss weak or problem areas early on in the nurse's allocation or appointment to the ward so that the nurse is given a chance to improve. A nurse should not be criticized in a report unless the problem has been brought to her or his attention previously.

It is preferable for student nurses to be given their final progressive assessment during the last week of their allocation and not to expect them to return at a later date. Time should be allowed for discussion and the student allowed the opportunity to write comments on the report form.

The staff development and performance review system is being introduced to many hospitals. Time is set aside at least once a year for the sister or charge nurse to discuss with staff nurses and enrolled nurses how they are getting on in the ward and to give them the opportunity to talk about their job, their contribution and their strengths and weaknesses. It is a two-way process with free and open discussion of the individual's progress. It is an opportunity to improve the effectiveness of the staff nurses' and enrolled nurses' performance and to develop their potential. Difficulties and problems can be discussed, training needs identified and a plan of action made. If a staff nurse on a medical ward, for example, lacks confidence when caring for patients following myocardial infarction, through the unit nurse manager it may be possible to arrange a few weeks experience in a coronary care unit. On the other hand, if a staff nurse is showing potential in the training of learners this may be extended by giving her or him specific responsibilities in the training of students in the ward. This is an example of building on a strong attribute.

The date for an appraisal interview is arranged with the appraisee well in advance and must be fixed at a mutually satisfactory time.

The interview must take place in a quiet place without interruption, and the discussion should be free and open and of a two-way nature. The appraisal interview should always be looked upon as constructive and never destructive. A special form is provided to be completed by the sister or charge nurse after the interview, detailing the agreed plan of action and it is signed by the appraisee, after she or he has been given the opportunity to read and discuss the completed form. It is then counter-signed by the line manager.

Training needs of others

There are others in the ward who rely on the sister or charge nurse for certain training needs from time to time. These include patients and relatives. Many patients have training needs, including learning to overcome a disability before being discharged back to the community (see Chapter 9). This will take place through rehabilitation either in the ward with the involvement of other health care workers, together with nurses and doctors, or in a special rehabilitation unit. Such units which exist for patients following such problems as injuries to spine, brain, eyes, hands, or legs, or after cerebrovascular accident, burns or amputation, to mention a few. Patients and relatives may be required to learn more skills, e.g. drawing up and giving an injection, recording blood sugar levels, administering parenteral feeds. Time needs to be allowed for these skills to be developed through observation and then practice under close supervision.

Newly qualified and newly appointed doctors tend to rely heavily on the sister or charge nurse for guidance with their day-to-day duties and location of basic and special equipment. It is important to make them aware of ward, hospital and authority policies and procedures.

Topics for discussion

1. Learning objectives for wards are usually drawn up with the student nurse in mind, and the learning needs of the permanent staff can easily be neglected once the orientation period is over and the specialist nursing skills have been acquired.

Either for yourself or for one or two permanent staff members, review the learning experiences that have been available in the last two months. Are there any ways of improving the quantity, quality or range of experiences available?

2. Think about how you might develop a small questionnaire to ascertain the opinion of student nurses and other short-term members of the ward team, in relation to their experiences on your ward. Would such information be of use to anyone, and would any changes be likely to result from it?

References and Recommended Reading

Burnard, P. & Chapman, C.M. (1990) *Learning Nursing – Aspects of Nurse Education: the way forward.* Scutari, London.

Butterworth, T. & Faugier, J. (ed.) (1992) *Clinical Supervision and Mentorship in Nursing.* Chapman and Hall Medical, London.

Fretwell, J. (1982) *Ward Teaching and Learning.* Royal College of Nursing, London.

Hinchliffe, S.M. (ed.) (1986) *Teaching Clinical Nursing.* Churchill Livingstone, London

Horne, E.M. (ed.) (1990) *Patient Education Plus.* Austen Cornish, London.

Kenworthy, N. & Nicklin, P. (1988) *Teaching and Assessing in Nursing Practice: an experiential approach.* Scutari, London.

Morton-Cooper. A. (1985) *The Nursing Student's Handbook.* Blackwell Scientific Publications, Oxford.

Ogier, M.E. (1981) *Ward Sisters and their influence upon Nurse Learners.* Occasional Paper, Nursing Times 77 11 (April 2nd 1981).

Ogier, M.E. (1989) *Working and learning: the Learning Environment in Nursing.* Scutari, London.

Orton, H.D. (1980) *Ward Learning Climate.* Royal College of Nursing, London.

Reid, N.G. (1985) *Wards in Chancery.* Royal College of Nursing, London.

Thompson, B. & Bridge, W. (1979) *Teaching Patient Care – A Handbook for the Practising Nurse.* Education for Care Series, HM and M Publishers, Aylesbury.

UKCC (1986) *Project 2000: A New Preparation for Practice.* UKCC, London.

UKCC (1990) *Report of the Post Registration Education and Practice Project* (PREPP) UKCC, London.

Chapter 12

The changing role of the nurse and the legal implications in patient care

A nurse is a person who has completed a programme of basic nursing education and is qualified and authorised in her or his country to practise nursing. Basic nursing education is a formally recognised programme of study which provides a broad and sound foundation for the practice of nursing and for post-basic education which develops specific competency.

International Council of Nurses, Mexico, 1973

The changing role of the nurse

As the attitudes of nurses and the public change, and as medical and surgical specialization and technology expand, the role of the nurse must develop to keep abreast of these changes. Alterations in nursing education and practice take place in order to keep abreast of current trends and new techniques within the profession and have an effect on the role of the registered nurse.

The nursing profession is going through a major change – that of accepting full responsibility for its own professional performance and standards of care, no longer being dominated by doctors. The hallmarks of the nursing profession are that a register is kept of all practising qualified nurses, there is a governing body which controls and disciplines its members, all trained nurses are accountable for the care they give, or do not give, there is autonomy of decision-making, a specific body of knowledge and a code of ethics. Nurses must keep their knowledge and skills up-to-date (see Chapter 11) and as their role changes more academic qualifications, such as the Diploma in Nursing or completion of a post-basic course, are required if they are to contend with the increasing demands made upon them. In 1978 the Royal College of Nursing Working Committee on Standards of Nursing Care recognized the dilemma for nursing caused by developments in diagnostic and therapeutic medicine, which lead to a strain between the caring and curing roles of the nurses with its effect on nursing standards. It came to the conclusion that the profession has the responsibility to assess where it should concentrate its activity in the interests of patients, and that it should plan and control its own area of work.

Nurses must be able to prescribe nursing care in relation to the nursing needs of a patient, as opposed to the patient's medical needs, in order to control the provision of, and determine the standard of care given. It is generally accepted that this involves recognizing the total health needs of the patient within the family and community setting, and the ability of the nurse to meet these needs.

It is essential therefore, that nurses in hospital widen their horizons and look outward from the hospital ward, concerning themselves with not only what befalls the patients whilst in hospital but also what occurs in the context of the patient's social setting and what needs to happen when the patient goes home – especially as the emphasis on community care is increasing, the trend being to keep people in the community for as long as possible.

The whole approach is towards the patients and their families. This is a team approach rather than the sole responsibility of one group of health workers.

Nurses must be prepared to consider extending their skills if this will benefit patient care, and also to participate in professional activities, becoming members of their professional organization. As the nurse's role has expanded, it is now deemed necessary to make it mandatory that all nurses, and not only midwives, attend a refresher course and re-register periodically, in order to safeguard the public (see Chapter 11).

Extending the role of the nurse

As medicine becomes more technical and as junior doctors' hours are reduced, nursing is affected. The prime function of the nurse is to provide care for the patient. This is interpreted in different ways, depending on the patients' needs. Those who have had cerebrovascular accidents, for example, are usually very dependent on the nurses initially to meet all their basic needs. As they improve, however, and are being rehabilitated, they are encouraged to meet these needs themselves with the nurses at hand to guide, encourage and support. Patients who have been severely burned are very dependent on nurses and doctors in the first instance, requiring both fundamental and technical care, until they are at the stage of rehabilitation.

It is accepted that nursing is primarily a caring profession with an overlapping of some functions with that of other health workers such as the doctor, the social worker and the physiotherapist. As bedside medicine becomes more technical, trained nurses are encouraged to take on more and more skills such as taking venous blood, administering intravenous injections, and defibrillating patients.

Legally, individual trained nurses are personally accountable for their own practice as well as for maintaining and developing their knowledge, skills and competence. They are, therefore, directly responsible for their clinical decisions and actions. As the needs of patients and relatives change on account of developments in research and technology, it is essential that nursing practice actively extends and advances to meet these changes.

Guidance from the Department of Health on the extended role of the nurse has been withdrawn and trained nurses advised that the United Kingdom Central Council's (UKCC) principles for practice, rather than certificates for tasks, form the basis for adjustments to the scope of practice. In developing their role, it is suggested that all nurses use as a framework the following documents issued to each trained nurse by the UKCC:

(1)   Code of Professional Conduct
(2)   Exercising Accountability
(3)   The Scope of Professional Practice.

Whenever contemplating developing the role of the nurse, consideration must be given to the resources available. The enhancement of nursing practice should be limited to those skills which will improve the quality of patient care, rather than taking over tasks other health workers want to dispense with or because nurses see these tasks as a status symbol, portraying themselves as mini-doctors or technicians. If a nurse extends her role, but in so doing compromises current aspects of care, or delegates inappropriately to others, the quality of care will suffer and the trained nurse will be held accountable.

If trained nurses undertake duties for which they are not properly trained and are therefore not competent to perform, and an error occurs, they become liable for action against them. To avoid this situation arising, when new medical developments are being considered within the ward, such as the introduction of new equipment, new techniques, or research activities, the sister or charge nurse must insist that there is full nursing involvement and discussion with the doctors, the clinical nurse manager and themselves before any extra tasks for the nursing team are considered. This also includes extension of outpatient clinics and the treatment of day patients on the wards, and any other activity which has staffing implications, however small it may seem at the time.

Policies and procedures are laid down by the employing organization to protect patients, staff and the organization. It is essential that the sister or charge nurse brings the policy and procedure manuals, copies of which should be available in all wards and departments, to the attention of all staff, especially those new to the ward, and that all nurses adhere to these. All alterations or additions to the manuals must be conveyed to all staff. Policies and procedures must be up-to-date and sisters and charge nurses have a responsibility to draw to the attention of senior nurse managers any policy or procedure which is no longer valid or cannot be adhered to for any reason.

The rights of the patient

Consent for operation

English law states that no one may wilfully interfere with another's body without their consent. This includes medical, surgical and dental treatment, exploratory procedures and internal examinations.

Persons of 16 years and over can give their own consent but children under 16 years require the consent of a parent or guardian. If, however, a minor between 16–18 years is living at home in the care of his or her parents, it is advisable to consult with them too, although they have no power to veto the consent of that minor. Consent may be verbal, written or implied. In hospitals, however, it is the practice to obtain written consent on a special consent form. Before obtaining signed consent for a specific operation, investigation or treatment, the doctor involved is required to give an explanation which is easily understood by patient, parents or guardian, together with a description of other options available for the management of the condition for which the patient sought treatment in the first instance. The type of anaesthetic to be used, if any, must also be clarified at this time. The nurse has a responsibility to ensure that this is done. In the unlikely event of the sister or charge nurse obtaining the patient's signature, if a query arises from the patient this must be answered by the doctor before the patient signs.

Any patient may refuse to sign a consent form and this refusal must be reported. If the patient is unconscious or is suffering from a mental disorder and is incapable of giving valid consent because of this, the proposed operation or treatment must first be discussed by the doctor with a close relative of the patient. In these instances written consent is not essential but is usually obtained. In the case of an operation for sterilization or artificial insemination the consent of both wife and husband is usually obtained by the doctor and a different type of consent form is used for this purpose. There are also special consent forms to be used for medical or dental treatment of a patient who is unable to consent because of mental disorder and when treatment is to be given by a health professional other than a doctor or dentist. It is advisable in all these instances to refer to local policies and procedures to clarify the local agreement on these issues.

Wills and gifts

Only a person in sound mind can make a valid will. When a will is drawn up the signature of the testator (person making the will) must appear at the very end of the will. The signature is made in the presence of at least two witnesses, who must be present throughout the signing and who must then each sign in the presence of the testator.

When a patient wishes to make a will it is wisest if the sister or charge nurse does not become involved or allow any of the ward nurses to become involved. Legally, anybody can witness a will but in the ward the nurse may need to leave the bedside to attend an emergency just as the will is being signed. It is sensible, therefore, that the nursing staff are not involved. If it is deemed necessary for a will to be drawn up immediately, a member of the hospital administrative staff must be contacted at all times. The administrator will then arrange for the will to be prepared and witnessed.

If a patient requests to make a will and the matter is not urgent it is advisable that the patient's solicitor is contacted and an appointment made for him or her to see the patient. If witnesses are required this should be arranged with the hospital administration department.

If a patient leaves a gift to a nurse or a doctor in a will, or if a patient gives a gift and subsequently dies, the beneficiaries of the will may ask for the return of the gift, especially if it is of great value. This is acceptable practice as the law states that 'If a gift is made by a patient to his or her nurse or doctor, there is a presumption that pressure was brought to bear'. It is advisable that nurses do not accept gifts from patients or their relatives to avoid problems that may later arise (see Code of Professional Conduct, Appendix I).

Complaints procedures for patients and relatives

From time to time patients or relatives make a complaint against a nurse, or against the hospital and every nurse should know what action to take if a complaint is made. Many patients and relatives do not complain even when it is justified because of the fear of victimization. The Patient's Charter (1991) states clearly that any complaint about National Health Service services is to be immediately investigated by a hospital general manager or health authority chief executive and a full and prompt written reply made. Guidelines for the action to be taken if a patient or relative complains are laid down by the Department of Health and also by the employing authority. (Hospital Complaints Procedure Act 1985 DA(98)14).

When patients or relatives complain, many of the complaints, for example, problems with diet or misplacement of an article of clothing, can be dealt with straight away by the sister or charge nurse. The complaint should be handled with courtesy for if not dealt with satisfactorily it may lead to a further complaint. If the ward sister or charge nurse is not able to deal with the grievance the help of the clinical nurse manager should be obtained. If the complaint is of a serious nature, for example, assault of a patient or theft, it should be reported to the clinical nurse manager immediately and it then becomes a formal complaint. The patient must be informed of the action taken as must the patient's medical consultant. All complaints made by patients or relatives should be documented fully in the patient's nursing records as this will assist in following up the grievance if a further complaint is made. Statements must be obtained from all staff concerned if the complaint is of a serious nature, and must contain factual information only.

A patient or relative may wish to make a written complaint and should be advised to write to the chief executive. All written complaints are thoroughly investigated. In some circumstances the sister or charge nurse may advise the patient or relative to put a verbal complaint in writing. If the sister or charge nurse makes a complaint on behalf of a patient and goes through the correct channels of communication to the clinical nurse manager and gets no satisfaction, the next line manager should be approached. If the sister or charge nurse is still not satisfied the Health Service Commissioner or Ombudsman may be approached.

Accidents and incidents

Sisters and charge nurses have a responsibility for the safety of themselves, those in the ward team, and patients and relatives. This forms an important part of the orientation of new staff to the ward, with the sister or charge nurse being prepared to train and supervise staff. All employees are responsible for providing a safe working environment, promoting their own safety and that of others by taking care, following procedures and using equipment properly. Safety policies must be available in each department and be brought to the attention of all staff when first employed.

Prevention of accidents

All nurses must be aware of all hazards or potential hazards in the ward to patients, visitors and staff and take the action necessary to prevent accidents occurring. Some hazards may be rectified by taking the appropriate action such as moving an obstruction from a doorway straight away. Other hazards, such as defects in equipment or structures, should be reported to the appropriate department immediately, and a check made that action is taken. The sister or charge nurse has a duty to make all new staff aware of potential hazards to nurses within the ward, such as radiation in an oncology unit, and the policies and procedures relating to these. Other possible hazards should also be emphasized, including the lifting and moving of patients and the handling of certain drugs such as cytotoxic drugs. The Health and Safety at Work Act 1974 asserts that if staff are involved in patient handling their employing authority has a duty to ensure that they should not be exposed to risks likely to cause them injury. It is vital, therefore, that all employees are made aware of the policy and procedures for lifting, that they are given opportunities for training and regular review of practice.

Patients should be supervised adequately to lessen the risk of accidents occurring, but a balance must be maintained so that independent patients and those being actively rehabilitated are not overprotected. Patients must be given a certain degree of independence, depending on their physical and emotional state. This will be achieved if the sister or charge nurse actively encourages the nursing care for each patient to be reviewed frequently.

Action to be taken when an accident occurs

All accidents, however trivial, should be reported. Full documentation is necessary in case of a complaint or coroner's inquest arising at a later date, and should be completed at the earliest opportunity. In the case of an accident involving a patient, visitor or nurse, a special form for the purpose of reporting accidents is completed by the nurse concerned. This should contain all the relevant facts about the accident, stated clearly and concisely, and must include the number and location of nursing staff on duty at the time, the location of the accident, how it was caused and, in the case of the patient, a description of the patient's physical and emotional state before and after the accident. The accident form should also contain the nature of the injury, the personal details of the person concerned and a description of any apparatus involved. The doctor in attendance enters the details of injuries sustained and signs the form, together with the nurse reporting the accident. Names and addresses of any witnesses (avoiding other patients if at all possible) are included and if statements are required these are attached to the accident form.

Good documentation is vital as it may be necessary to recall the facts months or even years after the accident has occurred. Claims for injury must usually be dealt with within three years of the incident occurring. If the injury does not come to light until after that time the claimant must lodge a claim within the next year although a judge may waive this time limit. If an accident results in the death of a patient the case is referred to the coroner. The coroner's job is to determine all the facts and an inquest is usually held at which members of the nursing staff may need to be present. This does not mean that negligence or lack of supervision is suspected. It is essential, however, that the coroner has all the facts of the case which, in the main, will be obtained from statements and accident forms, hence the need for accuracy. All accidents should be reported to the clinical nurse manager as soon as possible. In the case of a patient being involved details are entered in the patient's nursing records, and the next of kin informed. Any equipment involved is retained for inspection. If the accident victim is a member of staff other than a nurse, the appropriate head of department is informed, who should make the required report.

Health and Safety at Work Act 1974

The Health and Safety at Work Act was introduced as a broad act to cover every hazard affecting health and safety at work. It gave trade unions and professional organizations the power to appoint safety representatives who have a right to inspect work premises, which include wards and departments, and to investigate accidents and potential hazards.

The act has increased the responsibility of sisters and charge nurses, making them accountable for ensuring that the ward is a safe environment for patients, visitors and staff, and that staff adopt safe working practices. The sister or charge nurse must make sure that policies and procedures are revised as necessary. They also have a responsibility to safeguard other staff who may enter the ward when there is a particular hazard such as a radiation hazard, or an infection risk when barrier nursing a patient. It is advisable for the sister or charge nurse to be aware of her or his health and safety representative.

Since The Notification of Accidents and Dangerous Occurrences Regulations 1980, all fatal accidents and accidents resulting in major injury arising within health service premises are reportable to the Health and Safety Executive Committee by the hospital administrator. It is, therefore, extremely important that accidents are reported as soon as they occur. Members of staff have the right to report accidents which involve them to their health and safety representative.

Untoward incidents are also reported to the clinical nurse manager who notifies the hospital administration department. These, too, are reported in written statements. Untoward incidents include occurrences such as loss of dentures or a patient's property, damage to a patient's property or disappearance of a patient. Incidents must be reported fully so that they can be properly investigated and, in the case of damage to a patient's property, the appropriate action taken to compensate the patient. It is advisable to write a dated and signed statement whenever an incident arises, even if not requested to do so by the nurse manager, and keep it in a safe place, as the sister or charge nurse or nurses involved may be called to give an account at a later date. It is impossible to retain the full facts in the memory.

The legal implications for the trained nurse

As the responsibilities of trained nurses become more extensive and as a legal awareness is growing amongst the public, it is essential that nurses are aware of the legal implications involved. As health care professionals, trained nurses have a responsibility and are accountable to their patients and relatives, their profession and nursing colleagues, society and to themselves.

All nurses owe their patients a duty of care and must therefore comply with the standards of care and professional codes of practice laid down by the profession. This means that every nurse must exercise those skills that are reasonably expected of a trained nurse when carrying out nursing duties.

If any nurse falls below this standard and the patient is harmed the nurse is seen as having been negligent and is legally liable. The same applies if nurses undertake tasks before they have developed the appropriate skills and competence. In English law if any nurse is found to be negligent and causes damage to a patient, the patient or the patient's family can sue the nurse or employing authority up to three years from the time the injury is known to have occurred or from the child's eighteenth birthday.

Safeguards for the trained nurse

There are certain safeguards which help prevent these situations arising. Firstly, all trained nurses have job descriptions which explain for whom and to whom each grade of nurse is responsible, the functions of the job and the extent and limits of responsibility. Job descriptions should leave no nurse in any doubt of her or his responsibility for patient care and all nurses should be encouraged to refer to them.

Trained nurses are responsible for the activities of the untrained members of the ward team and it is, therefore, of paramount importance that when delegating the trained nurse makes sure that the person who is to undertake the work is competent so that the safety of the patient is not undermined.

The sister or charge nurse has an obligation to see that all nurses in the ward comply with the policies and procedures. If a member of staff is known not to be complying, for example, in respect of the administration of drugs or control of infection, the sister or charge nurse must immediately take the necessary action to find out the reason. If a nurse persists in not observing a policy or procedure, disciplinary action may be indicated. If all nurses follow policies and procedures they should always perform as safe practitioners, ensuring that no harm comes to the patient.

All trained nurses have a responsibility to themselves, their patients and their colleagues to be always professionally up-to-date, improving professional knowledge and competence on a continuous basis. By being aware of changes and new methods and techniques it will help them to perform safely and competently.

It is vital that when nurses return to the profession after a break they are given a full orientation and induction. This should include familiarizing them with all policies and procedures and other relevant legal documents. Once they have taken up their post in the ward these must be reinforced by the sister or charge nurse. In some hospitals, in the absence of an induction programme, the responsibility for the orientation and induction becomes the responsibility of the sister or charge nurse. No nurse should ever be put into a situation for which she or he has not received proper training or orientation. This rule must be observed by sisters and charge nurses in relation to their staff in the ward.

Custody of drugs

All drugs should be stored in a locked cupboard and given only when prescribed, in writing, by a doctor. It is very unwise to administer a drug for which there is no written prescription unless local policy allows, e.g. laxatives, antacids etc. The ward sister or charge nurse is responsible for the storage and stock levels in her or his ward or department, and the drug keys must be held by the nurse-in-charge.

Controlled drugs

The supply, storage and administration of all controlled drugs, which are highly addictive and liable to misuse and abuse, is covered by the Misuse of Drugs Act, 1971, and the associated Misuse of Drugs Regulations, 1985.

Within the ward, the custody of controlled drugs is the responsibility of the ward sister or charge nurse, who is the person legally authorized to obtain, possess and administer these drugs. This responsibility is also passed on to her or his deputy in the absence of the sister or charge nurse. The sister or charge nurse is, however, responsible for ensuring that the ward or departmental stock of controlled drugs is correct at all times, that the receipts and outgoings of the drugs balance, and for reporting any discrepancies as soon as they become apparent. The ward sister or charge nurse is well advised to check the ward stocks of controlled drugs on a regular basis, according to local policy. The pharmacist is also required by law to check the ward stock of controlled drugs against the Controlled Drug Register at least every three months. The drugs are supplied only on the receipt of the special order book, signed either by the ward sister or charge nurse, or her or his deputy.

A dose or part of a dose may be destroyed on the ward, but a container or part container no longer required, or date-expired, must be returned to the pharmacy department for return to stock or for destruction. In either case an appropriate entry must be made in the ward Controlled Drug Record book, preferably by the ward sister or deputy, and the pharmacist. The new regulations allow the destruction, on the ward, of controlled drugs brought in by patients, but this must be done in the presence of the sister or charge nurse and the pharmacist. It would be prudent to record this.

Borrowing of controlled drugs from ward to ward should be kept to a minimum but, if necessary, an appropriate entry must be made in the record books of both wards concerned. This is usually carried out with the authority of the senior nurse manager, but varies according to local policy.

All drug record and order books must be kept on the ward for two years following the date of the last entry. This is a legal requirement for all drugs records, not only controlled drugs.

Nursing decisions and nursing records

When caring for patients trained nurses must be seen to take all reasonable steps to protect them, making decisions which are consistent with good nursing practice. If, for example, a patient is known to have suicidal tendencies and is accommodated in a room which is not easily observed, the sister or charge nurse may be held responsible if the patient does commit suicide. Nurses will be criticized if it is observed that a patient is depressed and talking of suicide and then injures himself or herself, if the observation of new symptoms has not been brought to the attention of the doctor in charge of the case. Cotsides are not always a safeguard for patients who are confused and are persistently getting out of bed and falling as their use may aggravate an already distressed patient. In some cases their use may precipitate serious injury if the patient climbs over them. They may, however, help to avoid injury. The nurses will be seen to exercise reasonable judgement if they decide the patient is safer in bed without cotsides, with the bed at its lowest position or, alternatively, sitting out of bed in an easy chair. The patient must be continually assessed and the nursing plan altered if necessary.

In each case there must be full documentation in the patient's nursing records (see Chapter 2) as, in the event of an action being brought against the nurse or the authority the inquiry may take place several years after the patient's stay in hospital. Trained nurses are accountable for the care they have given and this includes accurately and legibly written nursing records, dated, timed and signed by the nurse writing the report. Omissions in the patients' nursing records could suggest that care has not been given. All nurses should write in patients' nursing records on the assumption that patients may have access to them, emphasizing the importance of being factual and legible. Any alterations made to nursing records should be carried out in a proper manner so as to signify that these were not made after a complaint has been received. When alterations are made this should be done by putting a line through the error, and dating and initialling it. Errors should not be scored out or obliterated with gummed paper or correcting fluid, which may give rise to suspicion. The same principle applies to drug record books and drug treatment sheets.

All observations of a patient's mental state which have been reported to the doctor must be recorded, as must any action recommended or taken. Informative nursing records are a safeguard for the nurse.

If the ward is understaffed or the facilities are so poor that patient care is at risk, the sister or nurse in charge must report this to the senior nurse manager immediately, and in writing if necessary. If action is not forthcoming the complaint must be taken to a higher authority.

Confidentiality of nursing and medical records

All information about patients available to the nurse, both written and verbal, must be considered confidential and disclosed only to nurses, doctors and certain other approved health workers. The relationship between the nurse and the patient is one of trust and the nurse has a duty to respect the patient's confidence at all times. If the nurse is in any doubt at all about the confidentiality of any information it must not be disclosed. This can be a difficult decision to make when talking to patients' relatives and it is always wise to obtain the patient's consent. Patients may request that information about their illness is not given to their relatives and this wish must be respected. Maintaining confidentiality must always be emphasized with all untrained personnel in the ward, including ward clerks.

Enquiries are often received from the police, the press and solicitors. These should be channelled through the hospital administration department. Clinical information required by the police must not be given without the consent of the doctor concerned who should provide the information and also decide whether it is unethical not to obtain the patient's consent.

In law there are instances when the nurse has a legal obligation to disclose confidential information. These include occasions when the patient has given consent, when requested by a court of law, and when assisting in the detection of a crime. The sister or charge nurse is, however, advised always to seek advice in these situations. If a patient has given permission for information to be given to a friend or relative who lives at a distance and that person enquires by telephone, the caller should be asked to call back if possible. This will ensure that the call is genuine. If the sister or charge nurse needs to inform a relative by telephone of an alteration in the condition of a patient, this practice is acceptable.

All patients' records, both nursing and medical, must be kept in a safe place in the ward, preferably in a special trolley or cupboard, away from access by patients and visitors to the ward.

Access to Health Records Act 1990

Patients have a legal right of access to information recorded about them in all manually held health records after November 1 1991, but not to see files on them prior to this date. The right of access is limited to the patient, a person writing on behalf of the patient and authorized by him or her to do so, the person with parental responsibility for the patient, a person appointed by the court to manage the affairs of a patient or, after death, the patient's personal representative.

Access to health records may be informal or formal. If informal, the health professional responsible for that episode of treatment may, on request, hand the patient his health record, but only the section he or she has compiled. Formal access is via the medical records officer, using the special request form, 'Application for Access to Health Records'. The Act applies equally to hospital and general practice records.

Access should be expected within 40 days and, if a formal request is made, a fee may be charged. If access is denied, a court order can be requested, although use of the hospital complaints procedure should be suggested initially. Corrections to the record by the applicant are allowed. If, however, the record holder does not agree with the correction a note of the applicant's views should be entered in the record.

Data Protection Act 1984

The Data Protection Act 1984 refers to automatically processed information about individuals, and regulates the use of that information. The Act stresses that data should be held only for the lawful purposes for which the hospital has been registered and that the information should be adequate and relevant (but not excessive), accurate, up-to-date, not kept longer than necessary and protected against disclosure or loss. Passwords allow access only to authorized persons, according to their roles and functions. It must be emphasized that all automatically recorded information is treated with the same degree of confidentiality as all other information about a patient. Under the Data Protection Act, computer records, including those compiled before November 1991, are open to scrutiny.

Storage of records

All nursing and medical records must be retained by the hospital for eight years after completing treatment or three years after the death of the patient. Secondary documents, e.g. observation records, may be sorted out after six years. Confidential records of all women who have had abortions must be destroyed after three years, but obstetric records and those of children must be retained until the child is 25 years old or for eight years from the death of the child or baby. In psychiatry, however, all nursing and medical records must be kept for a minimum of 20 years.

Duty rotas and records of property handed in for safe keeping are held for six years, but requisitions for stores and equipment are retained for only two years. These regulations are laid down by the Department of Health.

The rights of the staff

Grievance procedure

The local grievance procedure should be laid down in full as a policy and be drawn to the attention of all new staff. This procedure should be used sensibly by sisters and charge nurses. If a nurse within the ward has a complaint, it should be discussed in the first instance with the sister or charge nurse. If the sister or charge nurse has a complaint it must be discussed with the clinical nurse manager. When grievances or problems arise the person concerned should be prepared to talk to the supervisor or manager at the time as the problem can often be solved straight away. If sisters and charge nurses are approachable and understanding, many problems which arise for individual nurses can be effectively solved at ward level. If the problem is not resolved the local policy, which usually entails the persons involved approaching the next-in-line manager, must be followed. The correct channels of communication must always be used, rather than going straight to the most senior officer.

The grievance procedure is laid down so that issues affecting individuals or small groups can be resolved. If an issue which is not a personal one affects a large group of staff, it may be raised with the Staff Consultative Committee. This committee meets on a hospital basis and consists of representatives from management and from the professional organizations and trade unions.

Disciplinary procedure

If the sister or charge nurse shows self-discipline the nurse within the ward will follow this lead, and thus fulfil expectations of the public.

If a member of staff has to be disciplined, in the first instance this is done by the sister or charge nurse in a constructive, fair and helpful way (see Chapters 1 and 10). A disciplinary procedure is usually laid down to deal with persistent breaches of discipline, and serious offences such as being drunk on duty, drug offences or abuse of patients.

This procedure should be readily available to staff in policy manuals on wards and departments and the attention of all new members of staff should be drawn to it. In some hospitals members of staff are given a personal copy when they take up their post. Any nurse involved in a disciplinary procedure should be advised to consult her or his trade union or professional organization steward or representative straight away. As well as recruiting members and publicizing meetings, the steward or representative handles members' problems including grievance and disciplinary procedures. This may also include referral to the disciplinary committee of the United Kingdom Central Council.

The UKCC Professional Conduct Committee

The UKCC is responsible for producing rules governing all nurses in the United Kingdom. The Council also has disciplinary powers, being required by law to exercise this function through a special disciplinary committee which undertakes to:

(1) Protect the public who are vulnerable
(2) Maintain professional standards
(3) If possible rehabilitate the nurses concerned.

All cases of alleged professional misconduct originating from findings of guilt in the criminal courts, and allegations from the work situation (which must be proved) are referred by the police or the employer to the appropriate National Board. After obtaining further information the National Board Investigating Committee either closes the case, refers it to the Health Committee or to the Council's Professional Conduct Committee. Allegations of professional misconduct are judged against the UKCC's Code of Professional Conduct. The kind of offences dealt with include drug and alcohol offences, patient abuse, theft and dishonesty, assault and nursing offences. The UKCC has the power to remove names from the register of trained nurses if the nurse's conduct warrants this action. Once struck off the register a nurse is no longer able to practice. It is, however, possible in some circumstances to be restored to the register at a later date. Some nurses may be asked to serve a probationary period under supervision.

The UKCC health committee may consider offences which could occur because of a nurse's ill-health e.g. a depressed nurse who is working under very stressed conditions. Such problems are considered by this committee as opposed to the disciplinary committee.

Health and safety at work

The Health and Safety at Work Act was introduced to ensure that places of work are safe for employees and has been discussed earlier in the chapter. Any nurse who sustains an injury at work, however trivial, should report it to the sister or charge nurse who must ensure that medical advice is obtained and an accident report form completed. If the nurse refuses to get medical attention this should be entered on the form.

Ethical concepts

As developments in diagnostic and therapeutic medicine continue to take place, the conflict for the nurses between caring and curing becomes a greater problem for them. This is often intensified by the emphasis on the curing role of the doctors, especially in acute teaching hospitals. Ethical issues often arise, such as the confusion over when and when not to try to resuscitate a patient. There are other situations which can be equally concerning.

Other areas of concern and conflict occur when a patient asks the nurse about the diagnosis when the nurse knows that the doctor has been less than honest with the patient, when patients say that they do not want any more treatment or when patients' relatives are insistent that active treatment is continued at all costs even though there is no hope of the patient improving. It is vital that sisters and charge nurses identify these areas of conflict which might arise within the ward or department and are able and willing to support their staff at this time, as well as the patients and their relatives, through discussion and very careful explanation. It would be advisable to include the doctor too.

The UKCC Code of Professional Conduct (see Appendix I) affirms what the nursing profession expects of its practitioners by stating what standards the profession expects. If followed it should help nurses when called upon to make ethical decisions relating to patient care. Failure to meet the required standards may indicate misconduct on the part of the nurse. The ICN has also drawn up a code of ethical concepts which are applied to nursing (see Appendix III).

By having a code of conduct nurses are encouraged to question and challenge unsafe practices or anything which mitigates against the well being of the patient. These should be brought to the immediate attention of their nurse managers and, if appropriate, to their professional organization.

The code is designed to safeguard both the public and the nurse. The nurse can be asked to account for both acts and omissions of care if necessary. It is available to all nurses and is reviewed at regular intervals.

Advocacy

The Patient's Charter (1991) includes the right of the patient to be given a clear explanation of any treatment proposed, including any risks and any alternatives, before agreeing to the treatment. To make this goal achievable for the patient the registered nurse may need to act as an advocate for the patient as in other situations. The Code of Professional Conduct (1992) expects this in several of its clauses (see Appendix I).

The role of the patient's advocate is to defend, or speak up for, the patient and help him or her to make an informed decision, after ensuring that he or she has been given all the available information. The patient's final decision is supported by the advocate, even if this conflicts with the advice given by the specialists. The main function of the nurse advocate is to promote and safeguard the well-being and interests of the patient. Sometimes this will inevitably lead to conflicts with colleagues and other health care workers. Patients who are unable, because of various factors, to make informed decisions are most in need of an advocate.

The Patient's Charter also emphasizes that all patients have the right to refuse to be involved in research and the training of medical students without their treatment being adversely affected. In some instances the registered nurse may need to act as patient's advocate and defend this decision and make sure that it is honoured.

In order that conflict and confusion are minimized policy decisions made regarding each patient's treatment and management must be conveyed to the nursing team, who must also be informed of any change of policy. This responsibility rests with the sister or charge nurse. Any nurse who has difficulties in accepting certain decisions must be allowed the opportunity to talk this through with the sister or charge nurse, the doctor and, in some cases the hospital spiritual adviser. Decisions which are made on a team basis (see Chapter 8) also help to reduce the conflict for the nursing team.

Topics for discussion

1. Some of the most stressful situations for nurses arise because of ethical issues or conflicts. Review three recent stressful incidents in your clinical practice, and discuss why they were stressful and how the stress might have been reduced.

2. In some units, nursing history and assessment sheets and care plans are held by the patient's bed rather than in the sister's office. If this were done on your ward, what effect would it have on the content of the nursing record? Would any effect be detrimental or beneficial to the patient?

References and Recommended Reading

Access to Health Records Act 1990. HMSO, London.

Baly, M. (1984) *Professional Responsibility* (2nd ed.) Scutari Press, London.

Booth, J.A. (1983) *Handbook of Investigations*. Harper & Row, London.

Control of Dangerous Drugs and Poisons in Hospitals. (Aitken Report.) (1958) HM 58, 17.

Data Protection Act 1984. HMSO, London.

Graham, A. (1992) Advocacy: What the future holds. *British Journal of Nursing*.

Guidance on the preservation and destruction of NHS records. HM1673 and HM802.

Guidelines on confidentiality in Nursing (1980) Royal College of Nursing, London.

A handbook for nurse to nurse reporting. *King's Fund Project Paper* 21. (March 1979)

Health and Safety at Work, etc. Act (1974). HMSO, London.

Health Services Management: *Health Service Complaints Procedure*. Health Circular HM6615 and HC185, (April 1981).

The Misuse of Drugs Regulations (1985) DA 86 09.

Murphy, C.P. and Hunter, H. (1983) *Ethical Problems in the Nurse–Patient Relationship*. Allyn and Bacon, Massachusetts.

Patients Charter (prepared by the Department of Health) (1992). HMSO, London.

Pyne, R.H. (1992) *Professional Discipline in Nursing* (2nd ed.) Blackwell Scientific Publications, Oxford.

Rowden, R. (1984) *Managing Nursing*. Ballière Tindall, London.

Spellar, S.R. (1976) *Law Notes for Nurses*. Royal College of Nursing, London.

Standards of Nursing Care: A Discussion Document (1979) Royal College of Nursing, London.

Towards Standards: A Discussion Document (1981) Royal College of Nursing, London.

United Kingdom Central Council (1992). *Code of Professional Conduct for the Nurse, Midwife and Health Visitor*. (3rd ed.) UKCC, London.

United Kingdom Central Council (1989). *Exercising Accountability*. UKCC, London.

United Kingdom Central Council, (1992). *The Scope of Professional Practice*. UKCC, London.

United Kingdom Central Council, (1991). '... with a view to removal from the register ... an explanation of the system for considering complaints against registered nurses, midwives and health visitors which call into question their appropriateness to practice.' UKCC, London.

The Ward Sister's Survival Guide (1990). The Professional Development Series, The Professional Nurse. Austen Cornish Publishers Ltd., London.

Young, A. (1981) *Legal Problems in Nursing Practice*. Harper & Row, London.

Appendix I
Code of Professional Conduct for the Nurse, Midwife and Health Visitor (3rd Edition, 1992)

Each registered nurse, midwife and health visitor shall act, at all times, in such a manner as to:

- safeguard and promote the interests of individual patients and clients;
- serve the interests of society;
- justify public trust and confidence and
- uphold and enhance the good standing and reputation of the professions.

As a registered nurse, midwife or health visitor, you are personally accountable for your practice and, in the exercise of your professional accountability, must:

(1) act always in such a manner as to promote and safeguard the interests and well-being of patients and clients;

(2) ensure that no action or omission on your part, or within your sphere of responsibility, is detrimental to the interests, condition or safety of patients and clients;

(3) maintain and improve your professional knowledge and competence;

(4) acknowledge any limitations in your knowledge and competence and decline any duties or responsibilities unless able to perform them in a safe and skilled manner;

(5) work in an open and co-operative manner with patients, clients and their families, foster their independence and recognise and respect their involvement in the planning and delivery of care;

(6) work in a collaborative and co-operative manner with health care professionals and others involved in providing care, and recognise and respect their particular contributions within the care team;

(7) recognise and respect the uniqueness and dignity of each patient and client, and respond to their need for care, irrespective of their

ethnic origin, religious beliefs, personal attributes, the nature of their health problems or any other factor;

(8) report to an appropriate person or authority, at the earliest possible time, any conscientious objection which may be relevant to your professional practice;

(9) avoid any abuse of your privileged relationship with patients and clients and of the privileged access allowed to their person, property, residence or workplace;

(10) protect all confidential information concerning patients and clients obtained in the course of professional practice and make disclosures only with consent, where required by the order of a court or where you can justify disclosure in the wider public interest;

(11) report to an appropriate person or authority, having regard to the physical, psychological and social effects on patients and clients, any circumstances in the environment of care which could jeopardise standards of practice;

(12) report to an appropriate person or authority any circumstances in which safe and appropriate care for patients and clients cannot be provided;

(13) report to an appropriate person or authority where it appears that the health or safety of colleagues is at risk, as such circumstances may compromise standards of practice and care;

(14) assist professional colleagues, in the context of your own knowledge, experience and sphere of responsibility, to develop their professional competence, and assist others in the care team, including informal carers, to contribute safely and to a degree appropriate to their roles;

(15) refuse any gift, favour or hospitality from patients or clients currently in your care which might be interpreted as seeking to exert influence to obtain preferential consideration and

(16) ensure that your registration status is not used in the promotion of commercial products or services, declare any financial or other interests in relevant organisations providing such goods or services and ensure that your professional judgement is not influenced by any commercial considerations.

Notice to all Registered Nurses, Midwives and Health Visitors

This Code of Professional Conduct for the Nurse, Midwife and Health Visitor is issued to all registered nurses, midwives and health visitors by the United Kingdom Central Council for Nursing, Midwifery and Health Visiting. The Council is the regulatory body responsible for the standards of these professions and it requires members of the professions to practice and conduct themselves within the standards and framework provided by the Code.

The Council's Code is kept under review and any recommendations for change and improvement would be welcomed and should be addressed to the:

Registrar and Chief Executive, United Kingdom Central Council for Nursing, Midwifery and Health Visiting, 23 Portland Place, London, W1N 3AF.

Reproduced with the kind permission of the UKCC.

Appendix II
Useful Addresses

Every effort has been made to ensure that the following addresses and bibliographical details are current and correct, but the Publishers will be most grateful for information regarding any recent changes, along with suggestions for new inclusions in future editions.

International Council for Nurses
37 rue Vermont, 1202 Geneva, Switzerland

UK Statutory Bodies

United Kingdom Central Council for Nursing, Midwifery and Health Visiting (UKCC)
23 Portland Place, London W1N 3AF

English National Board for Nursing, Midwifery and Health Visiting (ENB)
Victory House, 170 Tottenham Court Road, London W1P 0HA

National Board for Nursing, Midwifery and Health Visiting for Northern Ireland
123/137 York Street, Belfast BT15 1JB

National Board for Nursing, Midwifery and Health Visiting for Scotland
Trinity Park House, South Trinity Road, Edinburgh EH5 3SF

Welsh National Board for Nursing, Midwifery and Health Visiting
13th Floor, Pearl Assurance House, Greyfriars Road, Cardiff CF1 3AG

Professional Organizations, Trade Unions and Others

Department of Health
Richmond House, 79 Whitehall, London SW1A 2NS
Welsh Office
Crown Buildings, Cathays Park, Cardiff CF1 3NQ

Scottish Office
Dover House, Whitehall, London SW1A 2AU

Scottish Home and Health Department
St Andrew's House, Regent Road, Edinburgh EH1 3DE

Department of Health and Social Services, Northern Ireland
Dundonald House, Upper Newtownards Road, Belfast BT4 3SB

Department of Social Security
Richmond House, 79 Whitehall, London SW1A 2NS

King's Fund Centre
126 Albert Street, London NW1 7NF

Medical Research Council (MRC)
20 Park Crescent, London W1N 4AL

National Blood Transfusion Service
Moor House, London Wall, London EC2

Office of Population and Surveys (OPCS)
St Catherine's House, 10 Kingsway, London WC2B 6TP

Royal College of Midwives (RCM)
15 Mansfield Street, London W1M 0BE

Royal College of Nursing (RCN)
20 Cavendish Square, London W1M 0AB

Voluntary Organizations and Support Groups

The publications listed below are updated regularly and are a valuable source of information, containing contact addresses and telephone numbers.

The Voluntary Agencies Directory. National Council for Voluntary Organisations, NCVO Publications, London. (revised annually)

The Women's Directory (1991), The Parents' Directory (1989), The Health Directory (1990). All compiled by Fiona MacDonald, NCVO Publications, London.

Social Services Yearbook. Longman Group UK Ltd, Harlow.

The Hospital and Health Services Yearbook and Directory of Hospital Suppliers. The Institute of Health Services Management, 75 Portland Place, London W1N 4AN. (revised annually)

The Health Address Book: A directory of self-help and support organizations. The Patients Association, 18 Victoria Park Square, Bethnal Green, London E2 9PF.

Code for nurses – ethical concepts applied to nursing

The International Council of Nurses see the ethical concepts applied to nursing as follows:

The fundamental responsibility of the nurse is fourfold: to promote health, to prevent illness, to restore health and to alleviate suffering.

The need for nursing is universal. Inherent in nursing is respect for life, dignity and rights of man. It is unrestricted by considerations of nationality, race, creed, colour, age, sex, politics or social status.

Nurses render health services to the individual, the family and the community and coordinate their services with those of related groups.

Nurses and people

The nurse's primary responsibility is to those people who require nursing care.

The nurse, in providing care, promotes an environment in which the values, customs and spiritual beliefs of the individual are respected.

The nurse holds in confidence personal information and uses judgement in sharing this information.

Nurses and practice

The nurse carries personal responsibility for nursing practice and for maintaining competence by continual learning.

The nurse maintains the highest standards of nursing care possible within the reality of a specific situation.

The nurse uses judgement in relation to individual competence when accepting and delegating responsibilities.

The nurse, when acting in a professional capacity, should at all times maintain standards of personal conduct which reflect credit upon the profession.

Nurses and society

The nurse shares with other citizens the responsibility for initiating and supporting action to meet the health and social needs of the public.

Nurses and co-workers

The nurse sustains a cooperative relationship with co-workers in nursing and other fields.

The nurse takes appropriate action to safeguard the individual when his care is endangered by a co-worker or any other person.

Nurses and the profession

The nurse plays the major role in determining and implementing desirable standards of nursing practice and nursing education.

The nurse is active in developing a core of professional knowledge.

The nurse, acting through the professional organization, participates in establishing and maintaining equitable social and economic working conditions in nursing. (ICN, Mexico 1973 reaffirmed by the Council of National Representatives in 1989.)

Reproduced with the kind permission of ICN, 3, place Jean-Markeau, CH 1201 Geneva, Switzerland.

Index

Page references in italics refer to definitions in the Glossary

abstracts, *73*
Access to Health Records Act 1990,
  253–4
accidents
  report forms, 247–8, 256
  safety policy, 246–9
    action in case of, 247–8
    Health and Safety at Work Act
      1974, 247, 248–9, 256
    legal implications for nurses,
      249–50
    prevention of, 247
  see also emergency admissions
accountability
  legal, 13–14, 243, 249–50
  see also law, legal implications of
    patient care
activities of living model (Roper),
  nursing care, 99–100
Acts of Parliament *see* legislation
adaptation model (Roy), nursing care,
  99–101
administration, computers in, 64
admissions
  assessment of patients on, 102–6
  preparation of patients for, 137–58
    emergency, 153–5
    planned, 151–3
adolescents
  consents for operations, 244
  as patients, 149
advocacy, ethical concepts, 257–8
amenity patients, 156
anaesthesia, consent to operation and,
  244
annual leave entitlements, 133

anxiety
  hospitalization and, 137–45
    causes, 137–9
    manifestations, 139–41
    reduction of, 142–5
appliances, requisition of, 183–4
appointments, follow-up, continuing
  care and, 184–5
appraisal systems, 21–2, 89, 237–9
artificial insemination, consent forms
  for, 244
assessments
  continuous (staff), 21, 230–33, 238
  nursing process, 102–6
    computers in, 62
    identifying needs and problems,
      104–6
    observation, 104
    obtaining information, 102–4
audit, nursing *see* nursing audit

behaviour patterns, of ward sisters/
  charge nurses, 2–7
benefit forms, 170, 186–7
bereavement *see* death and dying
bias, *73*
  observer, *75*
Branch Programme, Project 2000, 221,
  231
Briggs report (1972), 1
budgeting, 65–9
  consequences for ward sisters/
    charge nurses, 68–9
  glossary, 73–6
  incremental, 66–7
  preparation of budgets, 66–8

sources of finance, 65–6
  zero-based, 67
bulletin boards, 36
burn-out, 200

care, of patients *see* patient care
care, duty of
  legal accountability of nurses,
    13–14, 243, 249–50
  see also law, legal implications of
    patient care
care planning *see* planning, nursing
    process
career development, 235–6
  see also promotion
case assignment *see* patient allocation
change
  implementation of, and morale,
    212–13
  taking on a new ward, 41–55
charts, data presentation and analysis,
    71–3
chi-square test, *73*
children
  consents for operations, 244
  health visitors and, 165
  nursing records on, retention times,
    254
  as patients, 148
  school nurses and, 166
classification, *73*
clinical decision-making, role of
    research in, 58–9
clinical nurse specialists, 170–71
clothing, patients, policy and
    procedure, 144, 155, 186, 198
Code for nurses (ICN), ethical
    concepts, 257, 265–6
Code of Professional Conduct
    (UKCC), 14, 81, 256, 257, 258,
    260–62
cohorts, *74*
colleges
  of nursing and midwifery, 46–7
    computerization and, 63–4
    Project 2000 and, 221

Common Foundation Programme,
    Project 2000, 221, 231
communication, 25–40
  barriers to, 27–8
  breakdown in, 32–3, 39
  bulletin boards, 36
  chain network of, 29
  with dying person, 169, 190–93, 199
    and family, 169, 173, 194–5, 199
  effects of relationships on, 30–32
  forms of, 25–6, 39
  on hospitalization, 145–8
  for information gathering, 104
  open networks, 29–30
  unit meetings, 36
  ward meetings, 35–6
  ward reports *see* ward reports
  wheel network of, 28–9
  written, 36–8
community midwives, 48, 165, 167
  code of professional conduct, 260–62
  Nurses, Midwives and Health
    Visitors Act 1979, 220
  see also health care workers
community nursing services, 48,
    164–7, 177
  liaison with prior to discharge, 183
  see also health care workers
community organizations, informal,
    170
complaints procedures, for patients
    and relatives, 245–6
computers
  Data Protection Act 1984, 254
  in nursing, 61–4
    glossary, 73–6
conduct
  codes of
    ICN code for nurses, 257, 265–6
    UKCC Code of Professional
      Conduct, 14, 81, 256, 257, 258,
      260–62
  misconduct *see* disciplinary
    procedures
confidentiality
  of records, 63, 252–4

Access to Health Records Act 1990, 253–4
Data Protection Act 1984, 254
consents, for operations, by patients, 244–5
consultant nurses, 48
consultants, 48
   in multidisciplinary teams, 162–4
   ward rounds, 163–4, 177
continuing care, 178–203
   discharge against medical advice, 189
   of dying patient and family, 169, 173, 189–98
   planning discharge of patient, 178–89, 202
   on transfer of patient, 187–8
continuous assessments (staff), 21, 230–33, 238
control groups, 74
coroners, role in cases of accidental death, 248
counselling, 19–20, 23, 198
   by hospital social workers, 169, 194
   by spiritual advisers, 172–3, 194
courtesy patients, 156
Credit Accumulation and Transfer Scheme (CATS), 237
criteria for care, nurse manpower planning, 86
criteria statements, in quality measurement, 91–4

data
   presentation and analysis, 69–73
      glossary, 73–6
data base, 74
Data Protection Act 1984, 254
death and dying
   accidental death
      coroner's role, 248
      notification regulations, 248–9
   collection of personal effects, 198
   continuing care, of patient and family, 169, 173, 184, 189–98
   registration of death, 197

religious and cultural beliefs, 194
   stages to acceptance of, 192
   support for nursing teams, 199–201
   undertakers, 197
decision-making
   consistency in, 5, 22–3
   nursing decisions, legal implications, 251–2
   patients' involvement in, 107–8
   role of research in, 58–9
delegation, 11–14, 17, 22–3
   functional, 13
   legal accountability, 13–14, 250
   training and, 20
demographic data, 74
Department of Social Security, benefits and financial assistance, 170
departments
   interdepartmental conflict, 33
   personnel familiarization, 50–51
dependent variables, 74
diagrams, data presentation and analysis, 71–3
dieticians, 174
diets, in nursing care, serving meals, 16–17
direct costs, 74
discharge
   against medical advice, 189
   planning of, 178–89, 202
      benefit forms, 186–7
      clothing, 186
      follow-up appointments, 184–5
      GP's letter, 185–6
      liaising with health care workers, 183–4
      liaising with relatives, 182–3
      medical certificates, 186–7
      patient teaching, 180–82
      prescriptions and dressings, 185
      suitcases, 186
      transport, 184
      valuables, 186
disciplinary procedures, 21–2, 213, 255–6

distance learning, 64
district nurses, 48, 164–5, 167, 177
  see also health care workers
drugs
  custody of, 250–51
    controlled drugs, 251
  patients' own, 153, 251
    computers and, 62
    on discharge of patient, 185, 187
  safety policies and, 247
duty of care, legal accountability of
    nurses, 13–14, 243, 249–50
duty rotas
  hostility between shifts,
    communication breakdowns,
    32
  planning, 119, 128–34, 135
    holidays, 133
    ward rounds and, 163
  records storage, 254

education *see* teaching and training
emergency admissions, 153–4
  clothing and personal belongings,
    155
  informing relatives and friends,
    154–5
enrolled nurses
  code for, ethical concepts, 257,
    265–6
  code of professional conduct, 81,
    256, 257, 258, 260–62
  competencies, 45–6
  Nurses, Midwives and Health
    Visitors Act 1979, 220
  performance review system, 238
  Project 2000, 221
  ward teaching, 223–4
  see also ward nursing teams
environment
  control of, 134
  see also safety policies
ethical concepts, 257–8
  advocacy, 257–8
  code for nurses, 265–6
  computers and, 63

experimental groups, 74

families, of patients *see* relatives
feedback
  in appraisal and discipline, 21, 23
  importance of in delegation, 12
  see also communication
finance, and budgeting *see* budgeting
first-level nurses *see* registered
    nurses
fixed costs, 74
food, in nursing care, 16–17
Framework of Audit for Nursing
    Services (Project 32), 78–9

general practitioner's letters, at
    discharge of patients, 185
gifts, practice and procedure on, 245
glossary of terms (computing,
    research, data analysis,
    budgeting), 73–6
graphs, data presentation and analysis,
    71–3
grievance procedures, 21–2, 255
  patients' and relatives' complaints,
    245–6
Griffiths Report, 42, 79–80

handovers, 33–5
hardware, 74
hazards, safety policy on *see* safety
    policies
health authorities, information
    exclusive to, 53–4
health care workers
  at ward level, 49–50
  in continuing care of the dying, 194,
    195–6, 198
  coordination with, 15
  liaison with prior to discharge,
    183–4
  multidisciplinary team approach,
    159–77
  see also specified personnel
health records *see* medical records;
    nursing records

Health and Safety at Work Act 1974, 247, 248–9, 256
Health and Safety Executive Committee, accidents reportable to, 248–9
Health Service Commissioner, role in complaints procedures, 246
health visitors, 48, 165, 167
  code of professional conduct, 260–62
  Nurses, Midwives and Health Visitors Act 1979, 220
  see also health care workers
Henderson's model, of nursing, 98–9, 100
hierarchy, status, effects on communication, 30–31
hierarchy of needs (Maslow), 98–9
holiday entertainments, 133
home nursing, 183–4
  night nursing services, 184
home visits, multidisciplinary team approach to, 176–7
Hospital Complaints Procedure Act 1985, 246
hospital social workers, 168–70, 194
Hospital Trusts, 42–3
hospitalization
  effects of and reactions to, 137–45, 157
    awareness of, 141–2
    causes of anxiety, 137–9
    emergency admissions, 153–5
    helping patients adjust, 141
    manifestations of anxiety, 139–41
    reduction of anxiety, 142–5
hospitals, information exclusive to, 52–3
hypotheses, 74
  null, 75

independent variables, 74
indirect costs, 74
individualized patient care, 113–16
inpatient care *see* patient care
inquests, 248

International Council of Nurses (ICN, code for nurses, 257, 265–6
interviews, types of, 74

job assignment, organization of patient care, 116–17, 135
joint appointments, 22, 47

Kron's summary of supervision, 16

law
  legal implications of patient care, 241–59
    accidents and incidents, 246–9
    changing role of nurses, 241–4
    custody of drugs, 250–51
    ethical concepts, 257–8
    nursing decisions and records, 251–4
    patients' rights, 244–6
    staff rights, 255–6
    for trained nurses, 249–50
  see also legislation
leadership, 8–9
  joint appointments and, 22
  styles of, 9, 208–211
  team morale and, 207–12
learning
  on ward, 217–20
    creating a learning environment, 23, 215–17
    learning opportunities, 228–9
  see also teaching and training
legislation
  Access to Health Records Act 1990, 253–4
  Data Protection Act 1984, 254
  Health and Safety at Work Act 1974, 247, 248–9, 256
  Hospital Complaints Procedure Act 1985, 246
  Misuse of Drugs Act 1971, 251
  Misuse of Drugs Regulations 1985, 251
  National Health Service and Community Care Act 1990, 81

Notification of Accidents and
Dangerous Occurrences
Regulations 1980, 248–9
Nurses, Midwives and Health
Visitors Act 1979, 220
'Working for Patients' (1989), 42
literature reviews, *74*

management, cycle of, 7, 8
management budgeting *see* budgeting
management structure, 42–4
nursing, 46
management systems, computerized,
64
managerial skills, 7–22
appraising and disciplining, 21–2,
213, 237–9, 255–6
caring and counselling, 19–20, 23,
200
communication *see* communication
coordinating, 14–15
delegating, 11–14, 17, 20, 22–3, 250
encouraging and supporting, 17–19
leadership, 8–9, 207–12
planning and organizing, 9–10
prescribing, 10
supervising and directing, 15–17
teaching and training, 20, 215–40
see also morale, of nursing teams
manpower planning, criteria for care
methodology, 86
Maslow's hierarchy of needs, 98–9
meals, in nursing care, 16–17
mean, *75*
median, *75*
medical certificates, 186–7
medical records
confidentiality of, 252–4
on discharge or transfer of patients,
187, 188–9
storage of, retention times, 254
medical teams, 48
role in multidisciplinary team
approach, 162–4
students, 48, 258
ward rounds, 163–4, 177

in ward teaching, 239
meetings
multidisciplinary teams, 175–6
unit, 36
ward, 35–6
mental disorders, patients with,
consents for operations, 244–5
mentors, role in training, 226, 228
methodology, *75*
midwives, 48, 165, 167
code of professional conduct,
260–62
Nurses, Midwives and Health
Visitors Act 1979, 220
see also health care workers
misconduct *see* disciplinary
procedures
Misuse of Drugs Act 1971, 251
Misuse of Drugs Regulations 1985,
251
mode, *75*
models, of nursing, 99–101
monitor, quality monitoring
methodology, 85–6
morale
of nursing teams, 204–14
guiding and disciplining, 213
implementing change, 212–13
leadership and, 207–12
responsibility and commitment,
212
multidisciplinary teams, 7, 159–77
clinical nurse specialists, 170–71
community nursing services, 164–7
consultants and medical teams,
162–4
ward rounds, 163–4, 177
home visits, 176–7
hospital social workers, 168–70
meetings, 175–6
occupational therapists, 174
physiotherapists, 171–2
radiographers, 175
specialist nurses, 170–71
speech therapists, 174–5
spiritual advisers, 172–3

National Board
role in cases of misconduct, 256
teaching programme, 220–37
National Health Service and
Community Care Act 1990, 81
National Insurance Hospital Inpatient
Certificates, 186
National Vocational Qualifications
(NVQs), 233
negligence
legal accountability and, 243,
249–50
see also law, legal implications of
patient care
NHS Management Executive, 78–9
NHS Trusts, 42–3
night nursing services, home nursing,
184
non-participant observation, 75
non-verbal communications, 26, 39
Notification of Accidents and
Dangerous Occurrences
Regulations 1980, 248–9
null hypotheses, 75
nurse mentors, role in training, 226,
228
Nurses, Midwives and Health Visitors
Act 1979, 220
nursing audit, 78–9
Phaneuf's, 88–9
nursing auxiliaries, ward teaching,
233–5
nursing care
organization of, 98–101, 134–5
Henderson's model, 100
Orem's self-care model, 100
Roper's activities of living model,
99–100
Roy's adaptation model, 101
prescribing, 10, 241–2
nursing education structure, 46–7
computers in, 63–4
see also teaching and training
nursing history, defined, 103
nursing personnel
management structure, 44–8

*see also specified nursing
personnel*; ward nursing teams
nursing policy and procedures
legal accountability and, 250
policy and procedure manuals, 53,
54, 244, 255
nursing process
for meeting patients' needs, 101–12
assessments, 102–6
computers in, 62–3
planning, 106–12
nursing records, 36–8
care plan implementation and,
109–10, 151
on discharge of patients, 187
legal implications, 110, 251–4
accident reports, 247–8
complaints procedures, 246
confidentiality, 252–4
retention times, 254
referrals to community nursing
services, 165, 166
on transfer of patients, 188
nursing research, 56–7, 235
computers in, 65
see also research, in nursing

observer bias, 75
occupational therapists, 49, 174
ombudsman, role in complaints
procedures, 246
operations, consents for, 244–5
Orem's self-care model, of nursing,
100, 101
organization, 96–136
control of environment, 134
see also safety policies
duty rotas, 119, 128–34, 135
nursing care, 98–101, 134–5
nursing process, 101–12
patient care, 112–17
patients' day, 97–8
role of nurse in charge, 9–10,
125–8
ward nursing teams, 117–25
orientation plans, 41–2

outpatient attendances, 150–51, 184–5
overhead costs, 75

PA Scale, quality monitoring
    methodology, 87
participant observation, 75
patient allocation, 122–3
    role of nurse in charge, 125–6
patient care
    legal implications of, 241–59
    lifting and moving, safety policy on,
        247
    organization of, 112–17
        individualized, 113–16
        nursing care, 98–101
        nursing process, 101–12
        patients' day, 97–8
        task/job assignment, 116–17, 135
    Patient's Charter 1991, 245–6
        advocacy, 257–8
    patients' rights, 244–6
        complaints procedures, 245–6
        consents for operations, 244–5
        gifts and wills, 245
    preparation for, 137–58
        adolescents, 149
        amenity patients, 156
        children, 148
        clothing and personal belongings,
            155
        courtesy patients, 156
        elderly patients, 149–50
        emergency admissions, 153–5
        outpatient attendance, 150–51
        patients' relatives, 145–8, 154–5
        planned admission, 151–3
        private patients, 156
        service patients, 156
        stress of hospitalization, 137–45,
            157
    relatives *see* relatives
    teaching, 239
        for discharge, 180–82
performance appraisal systems, 21–2,
    89, 237–9
performance review systems, 238

personal belongings, patients', policy
    and procedure on, 144, 155,
    186, 198, 249
personnel
    familiarization with, 42–51
    see also specified personnel
Phaneuf's nursing audit, 88–9
physiotherapists, 49, 171–2
pilot studies, 75
planning, 9–10
    nursing process, 106–12
        computers in, 62
        evaluation of care, 110–12
        implementation of care plan,
            109–10
police messages, following emergency
    admission, 154–5
policy and procedures
    legal accountability and, 250
    policy and procedure manuals, 53,
        54, 244, 255
population, 75
Post-Registration Education and
    Practice Project (PREPP),
    236–7
practice nurses, 166, 167
prescribing
    medical
        computers in, 62
        discharging patients, 185, 187
    nursing care, 10, 241–2
primary nursing
    organization of ward nursing teams,
        123–5
    role of nurse in charge, 126–7
private patients, 156, 186–7
probability, 75
professional conduct
    code for nurses, ethical concepts,
        257, 265–6
    code of, 81, 256, 257, 258, 260–62
professional development, 235–7
Project 2000, 44, 221–3
    supernumerary status, 222–3
Project 32, Framework of Audit for
    Nursing Services, 78–9

promotion
  professional development and, 235–7
  taking on a new ward, 41–55
    health authority information, 53–4
    hospital information, 52–3
    personnel familiarization, 42–51
    ward information, 51–2
prostheses, requisition of, 183–4

qualified nurses, competencies, 44–6
quality, 78–95
  definitions, 78–80
  quality assurance programmes
    measuring, 88, 89–94
    monitoring, 83–9
    setting up, 81–3
quality circles, 89
Qualpac, quality measuring methodology, 86–7

radiographers, 175
random sampling, 75
record-keeping *see* medical records; nursing records
referrals
  to community nursing services, 165–7, 183
  to hospital social workers, 168
registered nurses
  advocacy, 257–8
  code for, ethical concepts, 257, 265–6
  code of professional conduct, 81, 256, 257, 258, 260–62
  competencies, 45
  Nurses, Midwives and Health Visitors Act 1979, 220
  performance review system, 238
  professional development, 235–7
  Project 2000 and, 221
  re-registration, Post-Registration Education and Practice Project (PREPP), 236–7
  ward teaching, 223–4, 233
  see also ward nursing teams

relatives
  care of, when patient dying, 169, 173, 184, 189–98, 202
  communication with, 145–8, 154–5
    approachability, 4
  complaints procedures for, 245–6
  liaison with, prior to discharge, 182–3
  teaching, 164–5, 172, 239
reliability, of tests, 75
religious rites, at death, 194
reports
  on accidents, procedures for, 247–8, 256
  data presentation and analysis, 69–73
  see also medical records; nursing records
research
  in nursing, 56–61
  glossary, 73–6
research tool, 75
response rate, 75
Roper's activities of living model, nursing care, 99–100
rotas *see* duty rotas
Royal College of Nursing
  standards of care, 80, 81, 91, 92, 241–2
    dynamic standard setting approach, 90
Roy's adaptation model, nursing care, 99–101
Rush Medicus, quality monitoring methodology, 84–5

safety policies, 246–9
  action in case of accidents, 247–8
  Health and Safety at Work Act 1974, 247, 248–9, 256
  legal implications for nurses, 249–50
  prevention of accidents, 247
sample, 76
  random, 75
school nurses, 48, 166, 167

second-level nurses *see* enrolled
  nurses
self-care model (Orem), nursing care,
  100, 101
self-governing hospitals, 42–3
semi-structured interviews, *74*
service patients, 156, 187
shift-working *see* duty rotas
sickness benefit, claim forms, 186–7
social workers, 49, 50
  in continuing care of terminally ill,
    194
  hospital *see* hospital social workers
software, *76*
specialist nurses, 48, 170–71
speech therapists, 49, 174–5
spiritual advisers, 172–3, 194
  see also health care workers
staff appraisals *see* appraisal systems
Staff Consultative Committee, role in
  grievance procedures, 255
staff nurses *see* registered nurses
standard deviation, *76*
standards of care
  defined, 80, 90
  dynamic standard setting approach,
    90
  measuring, 89–94
  Royal College of Nursing, 80, 81, 91,
    92, 241–2
  see also quality
statistics
  presentation and analysis of, 69–73
  statistical significance, *76*
status hierarchy, effects on
  communication, 30–31
sterilization, consent forms for, 244
stress
  hospitalization and, 137–45
  of ward teams, 173, 200–1, 258
structured interviews, *74*
student nurses
  ward teaching, 215–16, 224–33
    continuous assessment, 230–33,
      238
    learning opportunities, 228–9

ward profiles, 229–30
supernumerary status, Project 2000,
  222–3
supervision
  as a management skill, 15–17
  Kron's summary of, 16
support workers, 48–9
  ward teaching, 233
  see also health care workers
symbolic communication, 3, 26

tables, for data presentation and
  analysis, 70–71
task assignment, organization of
  patient care, 116–17, 135
teaching and training
  by example, 3, 217–18
  and clinical decision-making, 58–9
  computers in, 63–4
  consistency in, 5
  Credit Accumulation and Transfer
    Scheme (CATS), 237
  distance learning, 64
  joint appointments, 22, 47
  learning environment, 23, 215–17
  nursing education structure, 46–7,
    63–4
  patients, 174–5, 239
    for discharge, 180–82
  Post-Registration Education and
    Practice Project (PREPP),
    236–7
  professional development, 235–6
  Project 2000, 221–3
  relatives, 164–5, 172, 239
  in ward, 20, 215–40
    enrolled nurses, 223–4
    learning environment, 215–17
    medical teams, 239
    methods, 217–20
    nursing auxiliaries, 233–5
    Project 2000, 221–3
    registered nurses, 223–4, 233
    student nurses, 215–16, 224–33
    support workers, 233
    ward reports, 34

see also safety policies
team meetings, multidisciplinary, 175–6
team nursing, 118–22
    role of nurse in charge, 125–6
    team leader role, 119–22
terminal illness, continuing care, of patient and family, 169, 173, 184, 189–98
training *see* teaching and training
transfers
    of patients, continuing care, 187–9
    of staff, taking on a new ward, 41–55
transport, for patients on discharge, 184
Trust Boards, 42, 46

UKCC
    Code of Professional Conduct, 14, 81, 256, 257, 260–62
    Code of Professional Conduct Committee, 256
    and national boards, teaching programme, 220–37
    principles for practice, 234
undertakers, 197
unit meetings, 36
United Kingdom Central Council for Nursing, Midwifery and Health Visiting *see* UKCC
unstructured interviews, 74

validity, of test measures, 76
valuables, patients', policy and procedures on, 155, 186, 198, 249

variables, 74, 76
    variable costs, 76
voluntary organizations, 170, 184, 198

walk round ward reports, 35
ward budgeting, 65–9
ward meetings, 35–6
ward nursing teams, 44–6
    creating high morale in, 204–14
    nursing auxiliaries, 233–5
    organization of, 117–28
        patient allocation, 122–3, 125–6
        primary nursing, 123–5, 126–7
        team nursing, 118–22, 125–6
    stress in, 173, 200–1, 258
    support for on death of patients, 173, 199–201, 202
    support workers, 48–9, 153, 187, 233
    in ward teaching, 20, 215–40
    see also enrolled nurses; registered nurses
ward organization *see* organization
ward profiles, for student nurses, 229–30
ward reports, 33–5
    wheel network communication and, 28
ward rounds, 163–4, 177
wards, information exclusive to, 51–2
wills, practice and procedure on, 245
'Working for Patients' (1989), 42
workload assessments, criteria for care system, 86
World Health Organisation (WHO), 79, 80